𝔐iniatlas

DR C. J. KEELING
THE MEDICAL CENTRE
VICARAGE ROAD
MICKLEOVER
DERBY DE3 0HA

Cardiovascular system

D0779069

Preface

To the Doctor:

This new edition of this Miniatlas Collection has been meant as a practical and essential support for your daily activities.

Its pocket size has been designed in order to make it easily transportable and to serve as a visual aid to explain to your patients diverse issues referred to the anatomy, physiology and pathology of the different components of the human body.

Illustrations are clear and precise and include all necessary references.

This edition also includes two annexes of unquestionable value: a list of tables with the normal values and data from laboratory tests and a directory of web pages related to the Miniatlas specialty.

We hope you find it as useful as we expect.

The Editor

Summary

ANATOMY/PHYSIOLOGY OF THE CARDIOVASCULAR SYSTEM
The cardiovascular system 12
Anatomy of the heart 14
Intracardiac flow 16
Blood supply to the heart, the coronary arteries 18
Myocardial fiber. Ultrastructure and contractility 20
Major blood vessels. Structure 22
The arterial system 24
The venous system 26
Normal blood flow 28
Venous return 30
Cardiovascular reflexes (baroreceptors) 32
Cardiovascular reflexes (chemoreceptors) 34
Normal blood pressure 36

HYPERTENSION
Causes
Hypertension 40
Essential hypertension 42
Secondary hypertension 44
Renovascular hypertension 46
Consequences
Hypertensive heart disease 48
Hypertensive encephalopathy 50
Hypertensive nephropathy 52
Hypertensive retinopathy 54
Hypertension, endothelial damage and atherosclerosis 56

ATHEROSCLEROTIC DISEASE
Risk factors for atherosclerosis
Age as an atherogenic risk factor 60
Family history and genetic defects 61
Diet 62
Dyslipidemia 64
Hypertension 66
Stress and personality 68
Tobacco use 70
Diabetes and the metabolic syndrome 72

Obesity... 74
Hyperhomocysteinemia... 76
Atherogenesis
Atherogenic lipoproteins 78
Atherogenesis, response-to-injury hypothesis........................... 80
Chronic endothelial damage................................... 82
Endothelial dysfunction 84
Proliferation and migration of smooth muscle cells.................. 86
Fatty streaks 88
Fibrous plaque formation...................................... 90
Phases in the development and expansion of
a coronary atheromatous plaque 92
Classification of atherosclerotic lesions.................... 94
Atherosclerosis and its consequences
Atherosclerosis, thrombosis and thromboembolism................. 96
Main vessels affected by atherosclerosis 98
Ischemic heart disease 100
Stable angina pectoris.. 102
Unstable angina pectoris 104
Angina pectoris, Prinzmetal angina 105
Chronic ischemic heart disease 106
Myocardial infarction 108
Subendocardial vs. transmural infarction 110
Morphologic progression of myocardial damage 112
Electrocardiogram and myocardial infarction.......................... 114
Complications of infarction, cardiogenic shock 116
Infarction complications, arrhythmias 117
Infarction complications, heart rupture 118
Complications of infarction, ventricular aneurysm
and cardiac thrombosis 119
Right ventricular infarction 120
Diagnostic triad of AMI 122
Carotid atherosclerosis 124
Clinical consequences of ischemic stroke................ 126
Iliac artery atherosclerosis 128
Intermittent claudication..................................... 130
Renal atherosclerosis 132
Renovascular hypertension 134

HEART FAILURE
Normal and hypertrophic myocardial fibers............................ 138

Types of heart failure 140
Left heart failure. Predisposing factors
Hypertension... 142
Valvular heart diseases: aortic stenosis.................................... 144
Valvular heart diseases: aortic regurgitation 146
Valvular heart diseases: mitral regurgitation........................... 148
Coarctation of the aorta 150
Left heart failure. Clinical manifestations
Left heart failure 152
Acute pulmonary edema 154
Right heart failure. Predisposing factors
Pulmonary hypertension.. 156
Chronic pulmonary disease 158
Valvular heart diseases: pulmonic regurgitation 160
Valvular heart diseases: tricuspid regurgitation 162
Right heart failure. Clinical manifestations
Right heart failure 164
Other causes of heart failure
Ischemic heart disease and heart failure 166
Cardiomyopathies as a cause of heart failure 168
Myocarditis and heart failure 170
Cardiac tamponade, constrictive pericarditis
and heart failure 172
Rheumatic fever and heart failure 174

DISEASES OF THE VENOUS SYSTEM
Deep venous thrombosis 178
Varicose veins of the lower limbs 180
Post-thrombotic syndrome 182
Pulmonary thromboembolism 184

OTHER CARDIOVASCULAR DISEASES
Aneurysms. Macroscopic aspect and localization................. 188
Diabetic angiopathy 190

References..192

Tables with laboratory reference range values
and other data of interest 195

Specialized web sites 207

Cardiovascular system
UPDATED EDITION

The first anatomical examinations, nowadays part of the history of medicine, highlighted the importance of the heart and the blood vessels. As far as physiology is concerned, the cardiovascular system plays a more crucial role than all the other body systems, since it is not only responsible for its own nutrition but also for that of the rest of the tissues.

In unicellular organisms, simple diffusion of substances is sufficient to maintain the dynamic balance that enables life. However, more complex structures such as multicellular organisms would be unthinkable without a system of oxygen and nutrient distribution.

Given the critical role of the cardiovascular system, it is easy to understand that anything that interferes with its good health will have an impact on other organs and systems.

In Western countries, the leading cause of death is associated with different conditions that adversely affect the normal functioning of the cardiovascular system; for example, the high prevalence of atherosclerosis interferes with blood flow and often affects the performance of the heart muscle.

Due to its unquestionable relevance and considering the great need to count on updated material on cardiovascular anatomy, physiology, disease and treatment, we want to offer you what we consider a very interesting scientific product. We hope to have created a work that is not only readable but also of high scientific rigor.

Anatomy/Physiology of the cardiovascular system

The cardiovascular system is sometimes just called circulatory system. It is made up of the heart –a pumping muscle–, and a closed system of vessels known as arteries, veins and capillaries. Via this closed circuit, blood is pumped by the heart and passes once and again through the different organs of the body.

The arteriovenous path of blood flow throughout the body starts in the left ventricle of the heart. From there, it travels through the aorta to all the arteries of the body to supply all the organs. After passing through the blood capillaries, blood flows towards the venous system and into the right atrium through the superior and inferior vena cavae. From the right atrium it is shunted to the right ventricle to reach the pulmonary artery and get into the pulmonary circuit; finally, it ends up again in the left ventricle to restart the cycle. The veins of the stomach, intestine, pancreas, gallbladder and spleen do not drain straight into the inferior vena cava as they previously pass through the portal vein towards the liver, and then empty into the inferior vena cava through the hepatic vein (1)(2).

The cardiovascular system

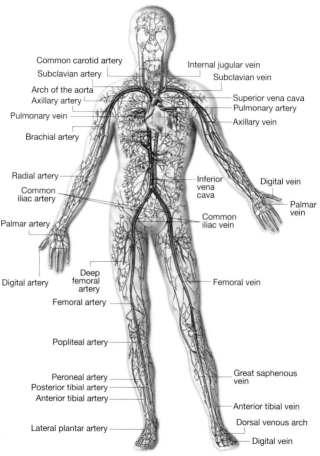

Common carotid artery

Subclavian artery

Arch of the aorta

Axillary artery

Pulmonary vein

Brachial artery

Radial artery

Common iliac artery

Palmar artery

Digital artery

Deep femoral artery

Femoral artery

Popliteal artery

Peroneal artery
Posterior tibial artery
Anterior tibial artery

Lateral plantar artery

Internal jugular vein

Subclavian vein

Superior vena cava

Pulmonary artery

Axillary vein

Inferior vena cava

Digital vein

Palmar vein

Common iliac vein

Femoral vein

Great saphenous vein

Anterior tibial vein

Dorsal venous arch

Digital vein

The human heart is an organ made up of muscle tissue; it has four cavities and its shape and size are similar to a closed fist. It lies in the mediastinum, or middle region of the thorax, immediately behind the breastbone (sternum) between the points of attachment of the second to sixth ribs. About two thirds of the heart mass are located to the left of the midline of the sternum, and one third is located to the right. The anterior aspect of the heart is almost completely occupied by the left and right ventricles, and only a portion of the right atrium is visible, which receives the superior and inferior vena cavae and the left auricle of the left atrium. The posterior aspect of the heart clearly shows the right and the left atria, the posterior portion of the left ventricle and a small portion of the lower right ventricle (1)(3).

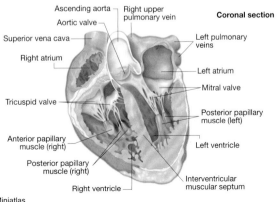

Anatomy of the heart

Anterior view

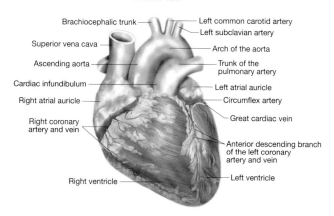

Brachiocephalic trunk

Superior vena cava

Ascending aorta

Cardiac infundibulum

Right atrial auricle

Right coronary artery and vein

Right ventricle

Left common carotid artery

Left subclavian artery

Arch of the aorta

Trunk of the pulmonary artery

Left atrial auricle

Circumflex artery

Great cardiac vein

Anterior descending branch of the left coronary artery and vein

Left ventricle

Posterior view

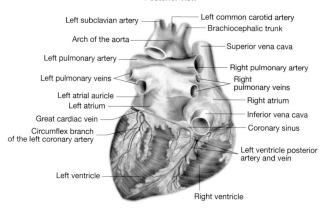

Left subclavian artery

Arch of the aorta

Left pulmonary artery

Left pulmonary veins

Left atrial auricle

Left atrium

Great cardiac vein

Circumflex branch of the left coronary artery

Left ventricle

Left common carotid artery

Brachiocephalic trunk

Superior vena cava

Right pulmonary artery

Right pulmonary veins

Right atrium

Inferior vena cava

Coronary sinus

Left ventricle posterior artery and vein

Right ventricle

Intracardiac flow is characterized by an almost independent operation of the left and right pumps. However, the movement of blood is well-adjusted thanks to the harmonic contraction of the heart, which is achieved through the heart conduction system. This system consists of the sinoatrial and atrioventricular sinuses and the Purkinje system.

In normal conditions, cardiac activity results from an impulse originating in a cell or group of cells that make up the pacemaker, and the transmission of that impulse to the atria and ventricles. When the electric signal reaches the contractile fibers of the heart, contraction is initiated. The term "cardiac cycle" refers to a complete heart beat or pumping cycle, consisting in the phases of contraction (systole) and relaxation (diastole) of both atria and both ventricles (2)(3)(4)(5).

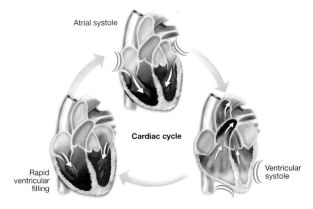

Atrial systole

Cardiac cycle

Ventricular systole

Rapid ventricular filling

Intracardiac flow

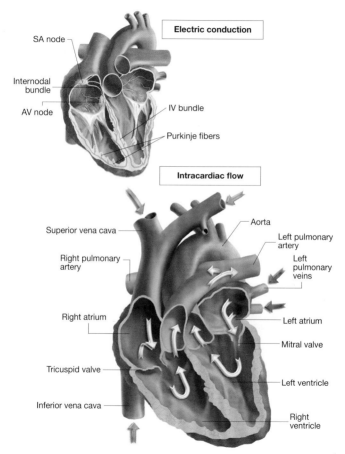

Electric conduction

SA node

Internodal bundle

AV node

IV bundle

Purkinje fibers

Intracardiac flow

Superior vena cava

Aorta

Right pulmonary artery

Left pulmonary artery

Left pulmonary veins

Right atrium

Left atrium

Mitral valve

Tricuspid valve

Left ventricle

Inferior vena cava

Right ventricle

Oxygen supply to the heart is performed by the coronary arteries and their branches. The coronary arteries originate at the root of the aorta, run along the heart surface and penetrate the muscle at a 90° angle. Like skeletal muscle, the myocardium compresses its blood vessels upon contraction. During systole, pressure inside the left ventricle is slightly higher than in the aorta. As a result, blood flow in the arteries that supply the subendocardial portion of the left ventricles only occurs during diastole. At rest, the heart pumps about 75% of the oxygen contained in every unit of blood volume. Only if blood flow is enhanced, it is possible to increase oxygen intake (1)(3)(6).

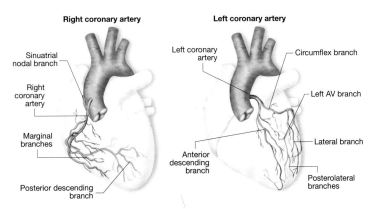

Right coronary artery

Sinuatrial nodal branch

Right coronary artery

Marginal branches

Posterior descending branch

Left coronary artery

Left coronary artery

Circumflex branch

Left AV branch

Lateral branch

Anterior descending branch

Posterolateral branches

Blood supply to the heart, the coronary arteries

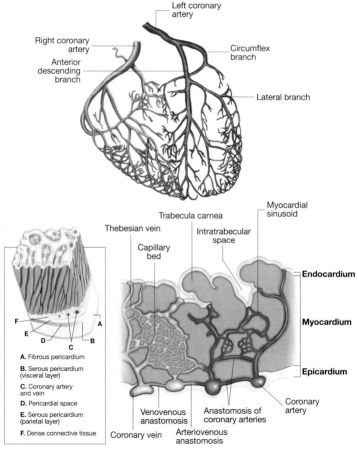

Left coronary artery

Right coronary artery

Circumflex branch

Anterior descending branch

Lateral branch

Trabecula carnea

Thebesian vein

Myocardial sinusoid

Capillary bed

Intratrabecular space

Endocardium

Myocardium

Epicardium

A. Fibrous pericardium

B. Serous pericardium (visceral layer)

C. Coronary artery and vein

D. Pericardial space

E. Serous pericardium (parietal layer)

F. Dense connective tissue

Venovenous anastomosis

Coronary vein

Arteriovenous anastomosis

Anastomosis of coronary arteries

Coronary artery

The heart is made up of a network of branched, striated muscle cells with a central nucleus. Each cell is limited by a plasma membrane (sarcolemma) and a mucopolysaccharide-rich basement membrane. Minute pinocytic vesicles are present along the whole cytoplasmic surface of the cells, which suggests an active participation of the sarcolemma in the transport of substances.

Nearly half of the cardiac fiber cytoplasm is composed of contractile fibrils, which are, in turn, formed by myofilaments arranged in parallel arrays. Fibrils are stretched structures resulting from repetition of the basic unit: the sarcomere. The myofibril structure contains two types of filaments: thick filaments made of myosin, and thin filaments made of actin. These two types alternate and cross bridge. Actin and myosin generate and regulate contractile strength acting in combination with other proteins: tropomyosin and troponin (2)(3)(5).

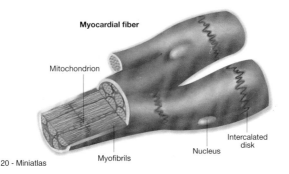

Myocardial fiber

Mitochondrion

Myofibrils

Nucleus

Intercalated disk

Myocardial fiber.
Ultrastructure and contractility

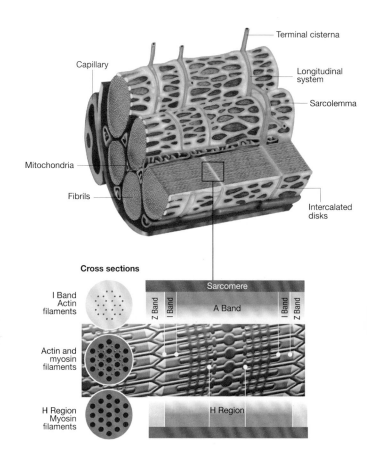

Terminal cisterna

Capillary

Longitudinal system

Sarcolemma

Mitochondria

Fibrils

Intercalated disks

Cross sections

I Band
Actin
filaments

Actin and
myosin
filaments

H Region
Myosin
filaments

Sarcomere

Z Band

I Band

A Band

I Band

Z Band

H Region

The vascular system is divided into two main types of vessels: *arteries*, which carry blood from the heart to the tissues; and *veins*, which collect blood from peripheral tissues and return it to the heart. There are two large circuits of blood circulation: systemic circulation and pulmonary circulation.

In systemic (greater) circulation oxygen-rich blood is distributed throughout the body and returns to the heart as desaturated blood. Conversely, in pulmonary (lesser) circulation, unoxygenated blood flows from the heart to the lungs, where it is oxygenated to return to the heart. Blood pumped by the left ventricle travels to peripheral tissues through the aorta. The aorta is responsible for supplying the head, the neck and the rest of the body. Thanks to a partial pressure gradient of gases, when the blood reaches the capillaries, it delivers oxygen to the tissues and picks up carbon dioxide. Desaturated blood from tissue capillaries is collected by the systemic veins that enter the right atrium via the superior vena cava and the inferior vena cava (1)(3).

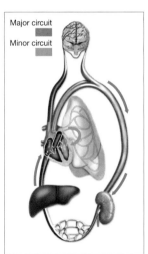

Major circuit

Minor circuit

Major blood vessels.
Structure

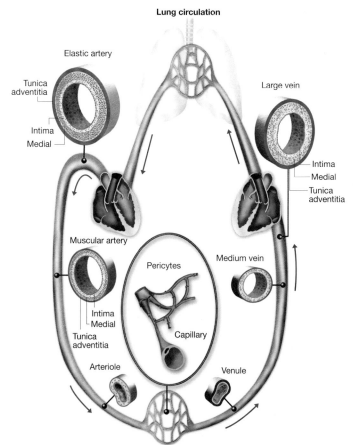

Lung circulation

Elastic artery

Tunica
adventitia

Intima

Medial

Large vein

Intima

Medial

Tunica
adventitia

Muscular artery

Pericytes

Medium vein

Intima

Medial

Tunica
adventitia

Capillary

Arteriole

Venule

Capillary bed

There is a system of blood distribution that originates in the left ventricle: the arterial system. This system is designed to carry blood from the heart to the tissues. Anatomically, it consists of contractile and elastic membranous ducts classified according to size into arteries –larger diameter– and arterioles –smaller diameter– which will later give rise to blood capillaries (tiny vessels specialized in gaseous exchange between blood and tissues).

Large arteries have very elastic walls to withstand high pressures. Arterioles are smaller vessels that distribute blood to all the organs and branch inside of them. As the arterial wall contains a large amount of smooth muscle, arterioles are also known as "muscular arteries"; for identical reasons, larger arteries have been termed "elastic arteries". Arterioles are also referred to as resistance vessels since, due to their small diameter, they are the primary site of peripheral resistance to blood flow. The last arteriole branching just before a capillary is known as precapillary arteriole (1)(3).

The arterial system

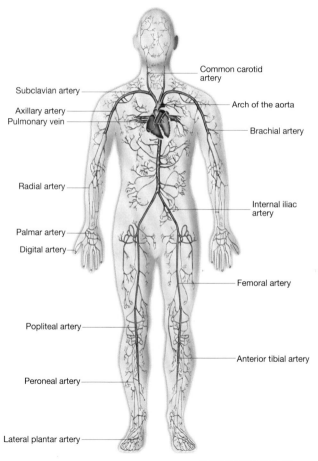

Common carotid artery

Subclavian artery

Arch of the aorta

Axillary artery

Pulmonary vein

Brachial artery

Radial artery

Internal iliac artery

Palmar artery

Digital artery

Femoral artery

Popliteal artery

Anterior tibial artery

Peroneal artery

Lateral plantar artery

The venous system is anatomically and functionally designed to carry blood from the tissues to the heart. From an anatomic viewpoint, the middle layer of a vein is thin compared to that of an artery. In physiological terms, veins are considered capacitance or reservoir vessels for they make up a large volume-low pressure system. Their high capacitance is due to wall distensibility. Veins are characterized by the presence of one-way valve systems which allow for blood flow towards the heart and prevent backflow. Based on diameter, vessels of the venous system can be classified into veins –the larger ones– and venules, which form as capillaries merge inside the tissues. Based on physiology, veins are classified as: collecting veins and venules; arteriovenous anastomoses also drain into the venules and, when they are open, they can shunt arterial blood directly into the veins (1)(3).

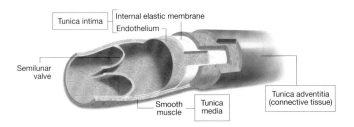

Tunica intima
Internal elastic membrane
Endothelium
Semilunar valve
Smooth muscle
Tunica media
Tunica adventitia (connective tissue)

The venous system

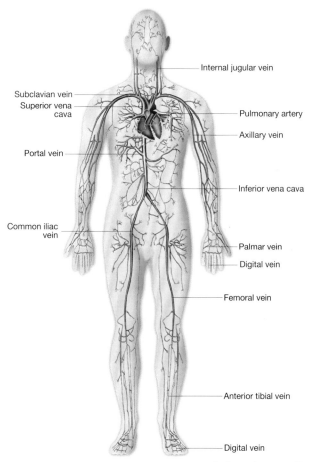

Internal jugular vein

Subclavian vein

Superior vena cava

Pulmonary artery

Axillary vein

Portal vein

Inferior vena cava

Common iliac vein

Palmar vein

Digital vein

Femoral vein

Anterior tibial vein

Digital vein

The cardiovascular or circulatory system allows for continuous blood flow in a virtually closed system.

The heart proper is a great muscular vessel with two pumps: a left one supplying the systemic circulation and a right one supplying the pulmonary circulation. Blood flow is given not only by the pumping action of the heart but also by the elasticity of arteries and compression of veins as a result of skeletal muscle contraction, aponeurosis and ligament tension.

Blood pressure and blood flow velocity are not uniform or constant but pulsatile.

The blood flow rate is governed by the physical principle whereby when fluid flows from an area of a certain surface transverse to another one, the flow rate decreases at the site of greater surface. Blood flow is slower in the arterioles than in the arteries since the addition of the transverse areas of all the arterioles exceeds those of the arteries. About one fourth of the blood is in the pulmonary circuit (lesser circulation), and the rest is in the systemic circuit (greater circulation).

Three fourths of the total blood volume are in the venous system, especially in the venules less than 1 mm in diameter. Under normal conditions, blood flow is laminar which allows for adequate circulation and a correct gas exchange at capillaries. In the presence of disease, flow can be turbulent, as in the case of valvular heart diseases or in arteries with atheromatous plaques (1)(3).

Normal blood flow

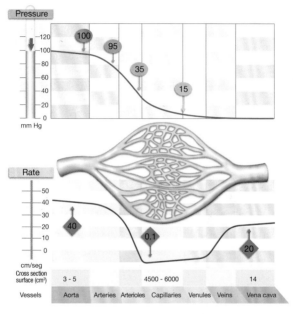

Pressure

120
100
80
60
40
20
0

100
95
35
15

mm Hg

Rate

50
40
30
20
10
0

40
0.1
20

cm/seg

Cross section surface (cm²)	3 - 5			4500 - 6000			14
Vessels	Aorta	Arteries	Arterioles	Capillaries	Venules	Veins	Vena cava

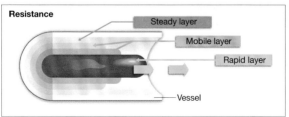

Resistance

Steady layer

Mobile layer

Rapid layer

Vessel

Venous return refers to the flow of blood from the venous system into the right atrium. To achieve this purpose, the circulatory system makes use of extravenous systems. The process of inspiration causes increased pressure gradient between peripheral and central veins by decreasing peripheral venous pressure. Every diaphragm contraction results in an increased volume of the thoracic cavity and decreased volume of the abdominal cavity. Thus, pressure is decreased in the thoracic portions of the vena cava and the atria, and increased in the abdominal cavity and abdominal veins. This change of pressures between inspiration and expiration behaves as a respiratory pump. The skeletal muscle pump acts by compressing the veins that run inside of it during muscle contraction. On the other hand, closing of the semilunar valves in veins prevents blood from flowing back upon relaxation of the skeletal muscle. The net effect of skeletal muscle contraction, together with the action of venous valves, is to increase blood return to the heart (2)(6).

Vein

Proximal valve closed

Skeletal muscles relaxed

Distal valve closed

Vein

Proximal valve open

Skeletal muscles contracted

Distal valve closed

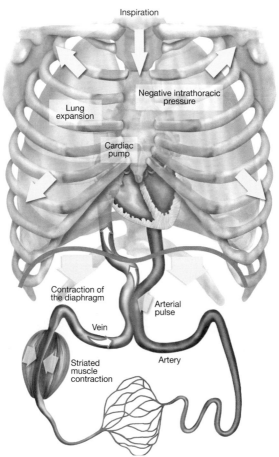

Inspiration

Negative intrathoracic pressure

Lung expansion

Cardiac pump

Contraction of the diaphragm

Arterial pulse

Vein

Striated muscle contraction

Artery

The baroreflex acts to compensate for or buffer any changes in blood pressure.

A rise in blood pressure stimulates baroreceptors and increases outflow rate. These baroreceptors are sensitive to changes in vascular wall tension. According to the law of Laplace, wall tension is proportional to the vessel pressure and radius (T=P.r); therefore, pressure changes stimulate receptors, and the greater the distensibility resulting from intravascular pressure, the greater the stimulus. Information of these receptors is received at the cardiovascular control centers, which determine a reduction in sympathetic tone and an increase in vagal tone.

As a result, and in response to the higher pressure, vasodilation occurs with decreased peripheral resistance. These phenomena cause blood pressure to return to normal values. Conversely, low blood pressure reduces arrival of impulses to control centers. Baroreceptors are free nerve terminals distributed in the adventitia of the major vessels walls and the atrial walls.

Afferent fibers ascend between both carotids to join the glossopharyngeal nerve. The efferent pathway of the reflex is formed by the vagus nerve and the sympathetic fibers that stem from the dorsal region of the spinal cord (2)(5).

Cardiovascular reflexes (baroreceptors)

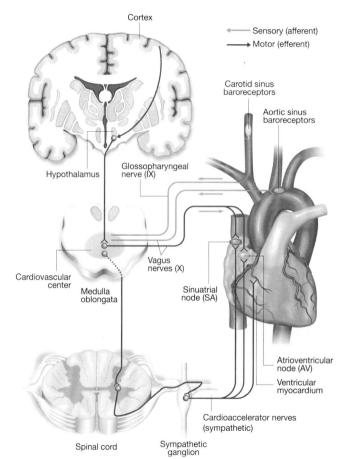

Cortex

Sensory (afferent)
Motor (efferent)

Carotid sinus baroreceptors

Aortic sinus baroreceptors

Hypothalamus

Glossopharyngeal nerve (IX)

Cardiovascular center

Vagus nerves (X)

Medulla oblongata

Sinuatrial node (SA)

Atrioventricular node (AV)

Ventricular myocardium

Spinal cord

Sympathetic ganglion

Cardioaccelerator nerves (sympathetic)

Chemoreceptors detect chemical changes in the blood and are classified, based on location, into central and peripheral receptors. Central chemoreceptors re located in the same regions as the cardiovascular control centers and act to control breathing actively. Peripheral chemoreceptors are found in the carotid body and the aortic arch.

Their afferent fibers join baroreceptor fibers and the vagus. Chemoreceptors are stimulated upon reduction of blood pO_2 or pH and increase of pCO_2. The response is not only increased pulmonary ventilation but also generalized vasoconstriction tending to increase blood pressure. Then, under these circumstances, chemoreflex response is only an alteration vasomotor tone. However, in severe hypoxia and hypercapnia, this vascular response may be accompanied by reflex tachycardia probably mediated by stimulation of central chemoreceptors. Chemoreceptor response to the decrease in pO_2 enhances the response of baroreceptors when these are inhibited due to a drop in blood pressure. This occurs, for example, when pressure decreases below 60 mm Hg, which can be easily evidenced by a section of chemoreceptor nerves in experimental animals (2)(5).

Cardiovascular reflexes (chemoreceptors)

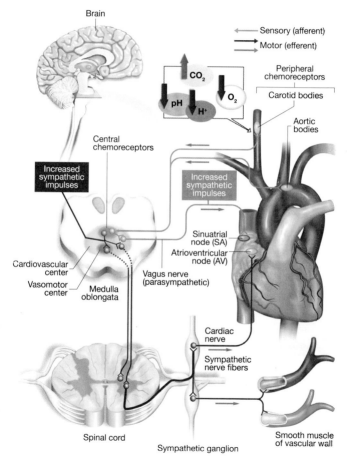

Brain

Sensory (afferent)
Motor (efferent)

CO_2
pH
H^+
O_2

Peripheral chemoreceptors
Carotid bodies

Aortic bodies

Central chemoreceptors

Increased sympathetic impulses

Increased sympathetic impulses

Sinuatrial node (SA)
Atrioventricular node (AV)

Cardiovascular center
Vasomotor center
Medulla oblongata

Vagus nerve (parasympathetic)

Cardiac nerve

Sympathetic nerve fibers

Smooth muscle of vascular wall

Spinal cord

Sympathetic ganglion

Pressure in the arterial system depends on two factors: cardiac output (CO) and peripheral resistance (PR). Pressure in the system is elevated when there is a cardiac output (CO) or stroke volume (SV) increase. Likewise, pressure rises as heart rate speeds up, which also elevates CO. Another physiological alternative to raise pressure without changing CO is to increase PR. The nervous system is the major regulator of peripheral resistance and exerts a tonic action on vessels, mediated by the adrenergic system.

In turn, central activity is modulated by the information received from peripheral receptors, baroreceptors and other peripheral structures. Peripheral resistance is influenced by humoral vasoconstrictor and vasodilator substances, as well as by local factors such as pO_2, pCO_2, pH and the accumulation of tissue metabolites. In normal conditions, and as a result of cardiac pulsatility, blood pressure measurement consists of two readings: systolic (about 120 mm Hg) and diastolic (about 80 mm Hg) (4).

Factors that determine normal blood pressure

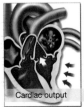
Cardiac output

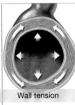
Wall tension

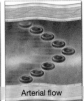
Arterial flow

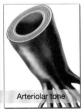
Arteriolar tone

Normal blood pressure

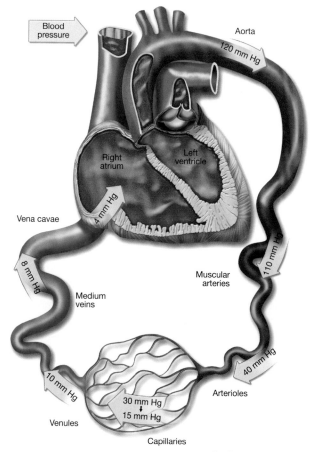

Blood pressure

Aorta
120 mm Hg

Right atrium

Left ventricle

Vena cavae
4 mm Hg

8 mm Hg

Muscular arteries

110 mm Hg

Medium veins

40 mm Hg

10 mm Hg

30 mm Hg
↓
15 mm Hg

Arterioles

Venules

Capillaries

Hypertension

Causes

Hypertension is defined as a chronic increase in systolic
or diastolic blood pressure. Hypertension diagnosis is established
when three readings, one week apart, confirm a systolic
pressure above 140 mm Hg or a diastolic pressure above 90 mm Hg
in an adult older than 18 years of age. When a systolic pressure
≤210 mm Hg or a diastolic pressure ≤120 mm Hg are confirmed, one
reading is sufficient for diagnosis. Based on etiology, hypertension can
be classified as: essential, primary or idiopathic hypertension, where
no cause is identified; or secondary hypertension, when associated
with some underlying condition, such as renal or hormonal
disorders (7).

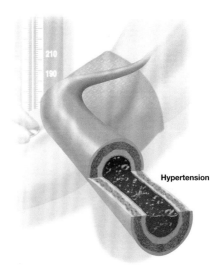

Hypertension

Hypertension

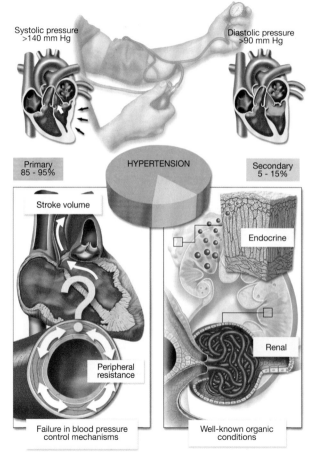

Systolic pressure
>140 mm Hg

Diastolic pressure
>90 mm Hg

Primary
85 - 95%

HYPERTENSION

Secondary
5 - 15%

Stroke volume

Endocrine

Peripheral
resistance

Renal

Failure in blood pressure
control mechanisms

Well-known organic
conditions

Arterial hypertension is, undoubtedly, the most frequent of the many chronic conditions that affect humans. Arterial pressure per se is nothing else but a figure that becomes relevant when increased, since the higher the systolic or diastolic pressure, the higher the morbidity and mortality of patients. This is so in all populations studied, in all age groups and in both sexes.

Hypertension is one of the most significant risk factors for cardiovascular disease and the main cause of heart failure, renal failure and cerebral infarction. In normal conditions, pressure is regulated by a number of feedback mechanisms.

Alterations in these regulation systems may lead to hypertension. When there is no identifiable cause or factor, it is termed essential or primary hypertension. This kind of disorder affects over 90% of patients with hypertension.

Secondary hypertension has, by definition, an identifiable etiology. Diagnosis of essential hypertension is basically established by exclusion, and only accepted when all secondary causes have been ruled out (8).

Essential hypertension

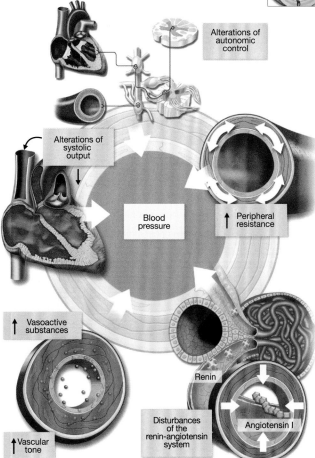

Alterations of autonomic control

Alterations of systolic output ↓

Blood pressure

↑ Peripheral resistance

↑ Vasoactive substances

↑ Vascular tone

Renin

Disturbances of the renin-angiotensin system

Angiotensin I

There is a small group of hypertensive individuals that present with identifiable factors and thus belong to the group of secondary hypertension patients. Secondary hypertension causes include coarctation of the aorta, Cushing's syndrome, certain drugs and hormones (amphetamines, oral contraceptives, estrogens, nonsteroidal anti-inflammatory drugs, cyclosporine, etc.), increased intracranial pressure, pheochromocytoma, primary aldosteronism, renal parenchymal disease and renovascular hypertension. All chronic nephropathies present with a higher incidence of arterial hypertension at some stage of the disease. Hypertension causes include chronic immunocomplex-mediated glomerulonephritis, chronic pyelonephritis secondary to infection, chronic interstitial nephritis, hereditary and radiation nephropathy, among others. A hypertension first diagnosed between 30 and 50 years of age can be the first manifestation of polycystic kidney disease. Only exceptionally, hypertension can be caused by obstructive uropathy and renal stones (8).

Secondary hypertension

Primary hyperaldosteronism

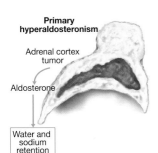

Adrenal cortex tumor

Aldosterone

Water and sodium retention

Vasoconstriction

Pheochromocytoma

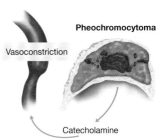

Catecholamine

Cushing`s syndrome

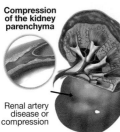

Unilateral pyelonephritis

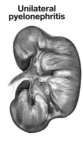

Polycystic renal disease

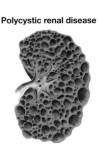

Compression of the kidney parenchyma

Renal artery disease or compression

Coarctation of the aorta

Luminal narrowing of one of the major renal arteries –or one of its branches– by 50% or more is responsible for 3-5% of hypertension cases. The two major causes are: a) atheromatous stenosis, more frequent in males and with an incidence that increases with age and a personal history of hypertension, diabetes or tobacco use, and b) fibromuscular dysplasia, which encompasses a heterogeneous group of lesions affecting one or more of the three layers of the renal artery. It is usually bilateral, and more common in women, especially younger than 30.

In renal hypertension, the factors that control blood pressure and are affected by the disease can be classified into three groups: 1) vasoconstrictor factors, especially the renin-angiotensin system; 2) factors that maintain urinary volume and salt homeostasis, and 3) vasodepressor agents.

These three mechanisms are closely interrelated. Increased renin secretion plays a critical role in renal hypertension secondary to unilateral stenosis of the renal artery (caused by atherosclerosis in 70% of cases). This situation is referred to as renovascular hypertension (9).

Renovascular hypertension

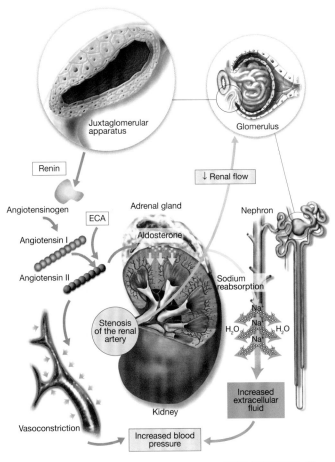

Juxtaglomerular
apparatus

Glomerulus

Renin

↓ Renal flow

Angiotensinogen

ECA

Adrenal gland

Nephron

Angiotensin I

Aldosterone

Angiotensin II

Sodium
reabsorption

Na⁺

H_2O

Na⁺

H_2O

Stenosis
of the renal
artery

Na⁺

Increased
extracellular
fluid

Vasoconstriction

Kidney

Increased blood
pressure

Consequences

Hypertensive heart disease may be asymptomatic and only suspected in the presence of an appropriate clinical context, with the finding of left ventricular enlargement revealed by ECG and ultrasound. Without adequate treatment, the effect of hypertension on coronary atherosclerosis leads to the development of a progressive ischemic heart disease. As a result of increased blood pressure the heart is subjected to increased workload and therefore, cardiac hypertrophy ensues. Increased pressure raises oxygen demand and accelerates atheromatosis, frequently triggering myocardial infarction. Cardiac hypertrophy is an adaptive response to pressure overload.

However, severe hypertrophy eventually results in myocyte injury, heart failure and dilated myocardium. Left ventricular failure is due to increased peripheral resistance to the extent that cardiac output can no longer be maintained despite the increased ventricular contraction as a result of muscle fiber elongation. There are often myocardial ischemic events that contribute to ventricular failure (9).

Hypertensive heart disease

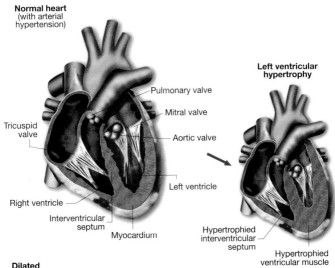

Normal heart
(with arterial
hypertension)

Pulmonary valve

Mitral valve

**Left ventricular
hypertrophy**

Tricuspid
valve

Aortic valve

Right ventricle

Left ventricle

Interventricular
septum

Myocardium

Hypertrophied
interventricular
septum

Hypertrophied
ventricular muscle

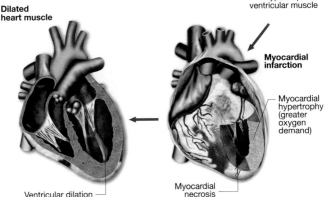

**Dilated
heart muscle**

**Myocardial
infarction**

Myocardial
hypertrophy
(greater
oxygen
demand)

Ventricular dilation

Myocardial
necrosis

Hypertensive encephalopathy results from an increase in blood pressure above the upper limit of autoregulation, the mean value of which may be 150-200 mm Hg in hypertensive patients. Autoregulation failure results in certain vasodilation areas, increased capillary permeability and edema. Signs and symptoms are by definition transient if blood pressure is promptly lowered to autoregulation levels; however, lack of treatment may lead to cerebral hemorrhage.

Cerebral hemorrhage is mostly associated with a history of hypertension and it is caused by the rupture of Charcot-Bouchard microaneurysms that occur at the bifurcation of small intraparenchymal arteries.

Although initial mortality is high, the process is not irreversibly catastrophic. Patients who survive initial hemorrhage have a relatively good prognosis (9).

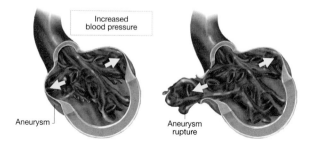

Increased
blood pressure

Aneurysm

Aneurysm
rupture

Hypertensive encephalopathy

Hemorrhagic infarction
(detail view)

Anterior
communicating
artery

Olfactory bulb

Aneurysm

Anterior
cerebral artery

Infarction

Subcallosal
artery

Internal carotid
artery

Middle
cerebral artery

Aneurysm

Posterior
cerebral artery

Basilar
artery

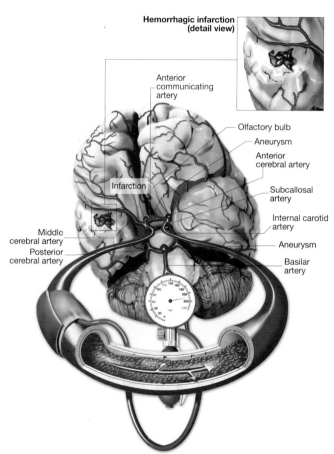

Kidney disease can be a cause of arterial hypertension, but it may also be a consequence.

In case hypertension is benign, the associated lesion produced on the kidney is known as hyaline arteriosclerosis. This form is known as benign nephrosclerosis and is very common in people older than 60 years of age. In younger individuals who suffer from hypertension or diabetes, it appears earlier in life.

Renal failure or uremia rarely occur. Vascular changes characteristic of benign hypertension involve increased renal vascular resistance and reduced plasma flow. Kidney size is usually reduced.

With adequate blood pressure control, renal function is preserved. This is not the case of malignant nephrosclerosis associated with malignant or accelerated hypertension. Previously normotensive individuals may develop this type of hypertension, though it is more frequent in patients with previous benign essential hypertension or chronic renal disease. Clinical evolution in these patients is morbid and usually results in a medical emergency.

Proteinuria is generally severe, although it rarely exceeds 5 g/day, and urinary sediment shows microscopic hematuria, gross hematuria or both, with hyaline and granular casts.

Kidney size is rarely reduced (9).

Hypertensive nephropathy

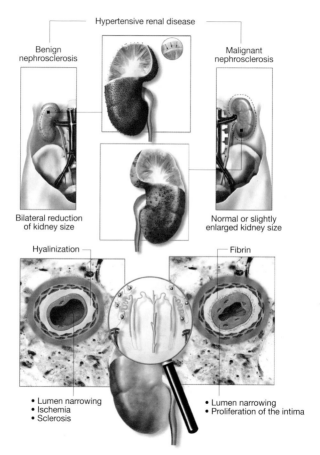

Hypertensive renal disease

Benign
nephrosclerosis

Malignant
nephrosclerosis

Bilateral reduction
of kidney size

Normal or slightly
enlarged kidney size

Hyalinization

Fibrin

- Lumen narrowing
- Ischemia
- Sclerosis

- Lumen narrowing
- Proliferation of the intima

Retinal lesions are frequent findings in systemic arterial hypertension and hypertensive encephalopathy. Hypertensive changes in retinal arterioles mainly consist of narrowing of their diameter.

In the case of acute severe hypertension, as well as in the initial phase of malignant hypertension, such changes primarily appear as focal spasms.

However, in chronic hypertension, arteriolar narrowing adopts a much more diffuse and slowly progressive pattern.

There are numerous classifications, but the one proposed by Keith, Wagener and Barker is the most widely used. Four stages are described: grade I retinopathy involves generalized narrowing of arterioles; grade II retinopathy also includes focal arteriolar spasms; grade III retinopathy presents, in addition to the above, "flame-shaped" hemorrhage, dot hemorrhage, spots and hard exudates. In grade IV retinopathy, papilledema is added to the above findings (9).

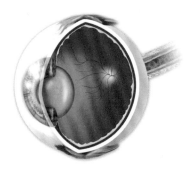

Hypertensive retinopathy

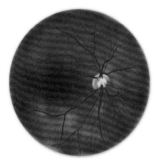

Grade 1
(Keith, Wagener and Barker)
Slight narrowing of veins

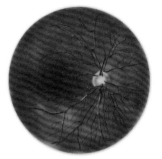

Grade 2
Moderate sclerosis with widened
light reflex and AV nicking

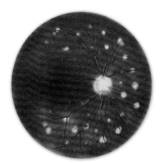

Grade 3
Exudates and hemorrhages,
sclerotic and spastic arteries
(silver wiring)

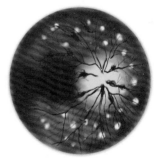

Grade 4
Papilledema.
Extensive hemorrhage
and exudates

Blood vessels are affected by hypertension. Vascular hypertrophy induced by pressure overload results from continuous stimulus and vasoconstriction, and is manifested by thickening of the internal elastic lamina and smooth muscle hypertrophy.

Hyaline degeneration (sclerosis and lipohyalinosis) is mainly observed in the renal afferent arterioles, although it also occurs in other organs. It extends from the subendothelial region to the tunica media via the deposition of eosinophilic material. Fibrinoid necrosis is a predominant anatomopathological finding in malignant hypertension. Vessel walls are damaged, showing necrosis and fibrin buildup. Cellular reaction may vary. Firstly, the endothelium is damaged, allowing plasma exudation to the media with tissue destruction.

Another lesion caused by malignant hypertension is endarteritis obliterans: the intima is markedly thickened by concentric collagen rings until the lumen is almost obliterated.

Hypertension is a significant risk factor for atherosclerosis, although its mechanism has not been completely elucidated. One of the possible mechanisms is mechanical stress which produces endothelial cell damage in high pressure areas of the arterial tree. Whichever the specific effect, it is clear that individuals with hypertension have a higher risk of death from atherosclerosis complications (10).

Hypertension, endothelial damage and atherosclerosis

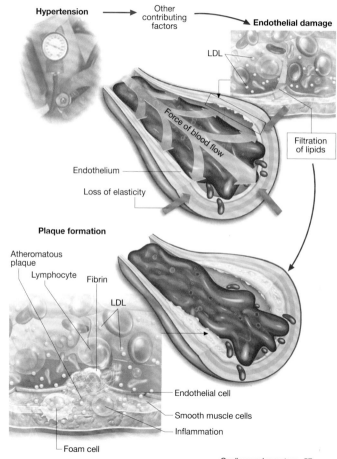

Hypertension → Other contributing factors → **Endothelial damage**

LDL

Force of blood flow

Filtration of lipids

Endothelium

Loss of elasticity

Plaque formation

Atheromatous plaque

Lymphocyte

Fibrin

LDL

Endothelial cell

Smooth muscle cells

Inflammation

Foam cell

Atherosclerotic disease

Age as an atherogenic risk factor

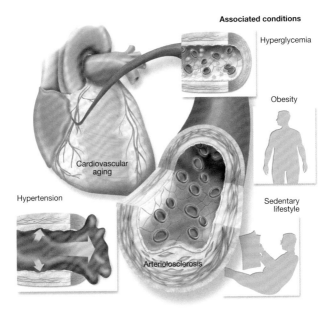

Associated conditions

Hyperglycemia

Obesity

Cardiovascular aging

Hypertension

Sedentary lifestyle

Arteriolosclerosis

Age is one of the non-modifiable cardiovascular risk factors together with sex and genetic factors. Cardiovascular risk is directly related with age, partly due to "aging" of the cardiovascular system itself, but also due to increased prevalence of other risk factors such as hypertension, diabetes, obesity, sedentary lifestyle, etc. All the cardiovascular risk scoring tables based on the prediction model of the Framingham Heart Study include age as one of the factors to take into account (11)(12).

Family history and genetic defects

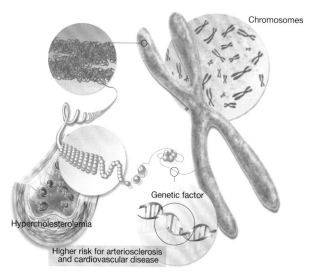

Chromosomes

Hypercholesterolemia

Genetic factor

Higher risk for arteriosclerosis and cardiovascular disease

It is not completely clear whether the correlation between a family history of heart disease and increased cardiovascular risk is only attributable to genetic factors or is a consequence of habits and lifestyle inherited from parents. However, certain genetic defects have been linked with increased cardiovascular risk, e.g. polymorphism of the fibrinogen beta gene or genotypes expressed as homozygous and heterozygous forms of familial hypercholesterolemia (mutation in the gene that encodes apo B:E specific LDL receptor). Most primary disorders associated with atherogenic dyslipidemias have an unknown molecular base and are classified as "polygenic" (11)(12).

Epidemiological studies carried out all over the world and in large population groups have determined that consumption of the typical "affluent diet" of industrialized countries is closely related to the prevalence of atherosclerosis.

The affluent diet is characterized by excess saturated fat and cholesterol –the two key nutrients for developing dyslipidemia–, as well as animal protein, refined sugars and sodium chloride, very low intake of vegetal fibers and a high total caloric value. This kind of diet is not only associated with atherosclerosis-related conditions (coronary heart disease, cerebrovascular disease, peripheral vascular disease, among others) but also to other conditions which sometimes coexist thus increasing the cardiovascular risk; examples of these are hypertension, type 2 diabetes and obesity (13).

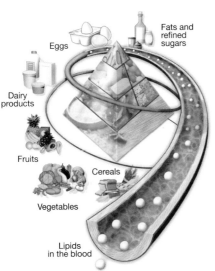

Eggs

Fats and refined sugars

Dairy products

Fruits

Cereals

Vegetables

Lipids in the blood

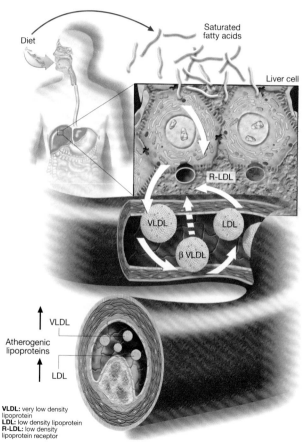

Diet

Saturated fatty acids

Liver cell

R-LDL

VLDL   LDL

β VLDL

VLDL

Atherogenic lipoproteins

LDL

VLDL: very low density lipoprotein
LDL: low density lipoprotein
R-LDL: low density lipoprotein receptor

It is currently accepted that cholesterol concentrations in plasma and, particularly, LDL-cholesterol concentrations, are major risk factors for developing CHD (coronary heart disease). This correlation has been well identified in epidemiologic/observational studies of important cohorts that have been prospectively followed. Evidence shows a continuous positive relation between risk for CHD and plasma LDL-cholesterol levels, and there is no defined "threshold" below which lower concentrations are associated with lower risk. These studies suggest that the cardiovascular risk increases by 2% every 1% increase in total cholesterol. In addition, the predictive value of HDL cholesterol levels as a risk factor inversely correlated with cardiovascular disease has been extensively confirmed. Recent data has evidenced that triglyceride values above 200 mg/dl entail a high risk for CHD and suggest that target values are below 100 mg/dl.

Lp(a) –lipoprotein (a)– is an independent risk factor for CHD. A relative risk for myocardial infarction 1.75 times higher if Lp(a) levels are over or equal to 300 mg/l has been reported (11)(12).

Dyslipidemia

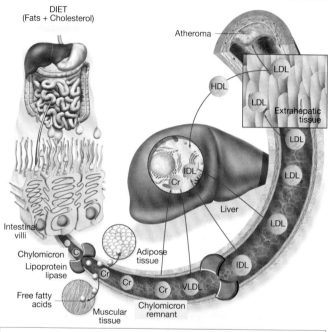

DIET
(Fats + Cholesterol)

Atheroma

HDL

LDL

LDL

Extrahepatic
tissue

LDL

IDL

Cr

LDL

Liver

LDL

IDL

Intestinal
villi

Chylomicron

C

Lipoprotein
lipase

Cr

Cr

Cr

VLDL

Free fatty
acids

Adipose
tissue

Chylomicron
remnant

Muscular
tissue

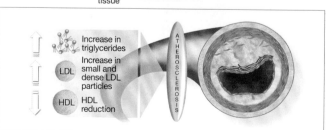

Increase in
triglycerides

LDL   Increase in
small and
dense LDL
particles

HDL   HDL
reduction

ATHEROSCLEROSIS

High blood pressure is directly related to the risk of cerebrovascular accident and myocardial infarction. Although hypertension is often associated to obesity and insulin resistance, the risk posed by hypertension enhances the risk presented by any of the other cardiovascular risk factors. The higher the blood pressure levels, the higher the risk of cardiovascular disease. A physiological and pathogenic observation reveals three hypertension-related disorders causing vascular damage: pulsatile blood flow, endothelial cell dysfunction, and vascular smooth muscle hypertrophy. High systolic pressure is known to be the main causal agent for these disorders; it entails a greater risk than high diastolic pressure (3)(5).

Muscular arterial wall

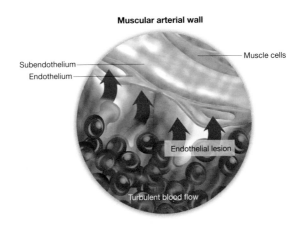

Subendothelium

Endothelium

Muscle cells

Endothelial lesion

Turbulent blood flow

Hypertension

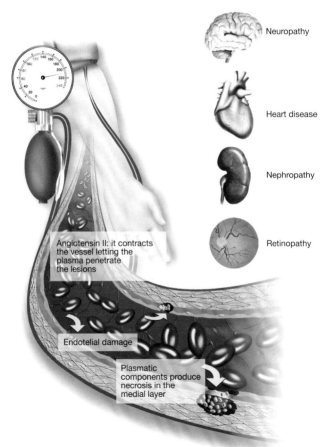

Neuropathy

Heart disease

Nephropathy

Retinopathy

Angiotensin II: it contracts the vessel letting the plasma penetrate the lesions

Endotelial damage

Plasmatic components produce necrosis in the medial layer

Faced to psychologically demanding chronic or stressful situations, the body response can be more subtle than the "fight or flight" behavior typically triggered by a dangerous or threatening situation. However, it can also be much more harmful.

Increased heart rate and blood pressure, together with higher levels of stress hormone (catecholamines and glucocorticoids) production may damage the endothelium.

As a result, it triggers a response which attempts to repair the lesion but may promote arterial wall thickening and accelerate the development of atheromatous deposits. This is mainly found in people of a type "A" behavior pattern (e.g.: irritable, impatient, setting excessive demands, dissatisfied with their accomplishments in spite of success) (13).

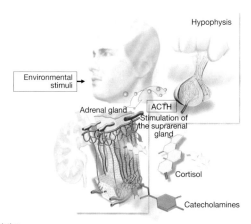

Stress and personality

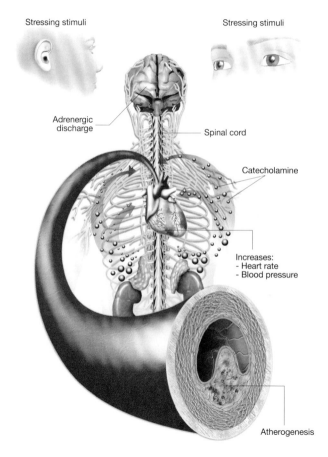

Stressing stimuli

Stressing stimuli

Adrenergic
discharge

Spinal cord

Catecholamine

Increases:
- Heart rate
- Blood pressure

Atherogenesis

Several studies have conclusively shown that smoking accelerates arteriosclerosis (hardening of the arterial walls) and the most common form of the disease, atherosclerosis, increasing the risk for coronary artery disease, cerebrovascular disease and peripheral vascular disease. The smoking habit raises LDL and triglyceride levels and reduces HDL levels; also, it promotes endothelial hypoxia as it raises blood levels of carbon monoxide. Furthermore, nicotine and other tobacco derivatives are toxic to endothelium and may cause its dysfunction. In addition, it promotes arterial vasoconstriction. In addition, cigarette smoking increases platelet reactivity and aggregation, and plasma fibrinogen concentration, which results in higher blood viscosity.

These negative effects of tobacco are directly related to the number of cigarettes smoked per day. Furthermore, passive smokers are at higher risk for coronary heart disease (13).

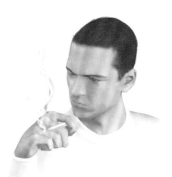

The smoking habit would accelerate the development of atherosclerosis.

Tobacco use

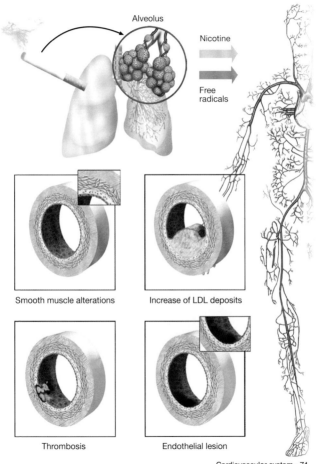

Alveolus

Nicotine

Free radicals

Smooth muscle alterations

Increase of LDL deposits

Thrombosis

Endothelial lesion

Coronary artery disease accounts for almost 75% of deaths in diabetic individuals. Although hyperglycemia is associated with small vessel disorders, insulin resistance promotes by itself the development of atherosclerosis even before it manifests clinically as diabetes. Diabetic patients show a marked impairment of the vascular smooth muscle and endothelial functions, as well as an increased leukocyte adhesion to the vascular endothelium, which plays a critical role in atherogenesis. The metabolic is determined by peripheral insensitivity to insulin. The syndrome's hallmarks are impaired glucose tolerance or diabetes mellitus, hyperinsulinemia, hypertension, central obesity, hypertriglyceridemia, low HDL levels, increase in small dense LDL cholesterol, and a procoagulant state. Patients with this condition are at high risk for cardiovascular disease.

The triad hypertriglyceridemia + HDL cholesterol reduction + increase in small and dense LDL particles promotes the development of atherosclerosis; some authors term it "atherogenic dyslipidemia" (3)(5)(14).

Diabetes and the metabolic syndrome

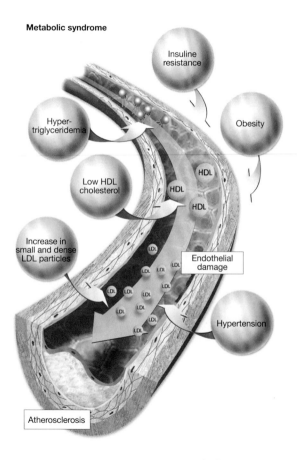

Metabolic syndrome

Insulin resistance

Obesity

Hyper-triglyceridemia

Low HDL cholesterol

HDL

HDL

HDL

Increase in small and dense LDL particles

LDL

LDL LDL LDL

LDL LDL LDL

LDL LDL

LDL

LDL

LDL

Endothelial damage

Hypertension

Atherosclerosis

Any degree of overweight appears to increase cardiovascular risk, and the higher the degree of obesity the greater the chances to develop other conditions predisposing to atherosclerosis (hypertension, atherogenic dyslipidemia, diabetes mellitus). The characteristic common to all these conditions is insulin resistance and the resulting hyperinsulinemia.

Obese individuals have a three-fold higher risk to develop heart disease as compared to subjects with a normal body mass index (BMI).

This association is even much stronger in cases of centripetal obesity where excess body fat is accumulated in the trunk, i.e. following the "android" pattern of body fat distribution. Both males and females with this type of obesity are at higher risk for developing vascular disease, particularly in the coronary and cerebral territories (13).

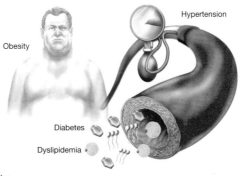

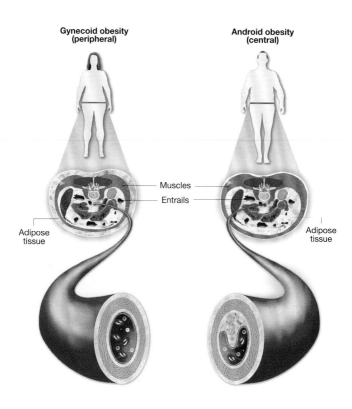

**Gynecoid obesity
(peripheral)**

**Android obesity
(central)**

Muscles

Entrails

Adipose
tissue

Adipose
tissue

The presence of congenital diseases of the homocysteine metabolism (with homozygous genotype) and very high serum homocysteine levels are positively correlated with premature atherosclerosis; these patients may have a myocardial infarction during the second decade of life. Homocysteine is toxic to endothelium: it has a prothrombotic effect, promotes collagen formation and reduces NO availability. In certain cases, patients suffer from moderate hyperhomocysteinemia; this disorder is positively correlated with risk for cardiovascular disease although not as closely as with the so-called major risk factors (11)(15).

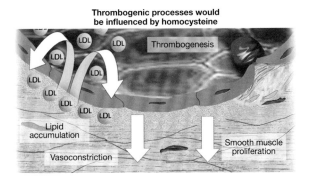

Hyperhomocysteinemia

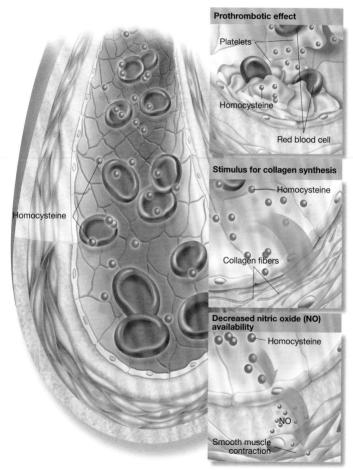

Prothrombotic effect

Platelets

Homocysteine

Red blood cell

Stimulus for collagen synthesis

Homocysteine

Collagen fibers

Decreased nitric oxide (NO) availability

Homocysteine

NO

Smooth muscle contraction

Homocysteine

Atherogenesis

LDLs are still considered the major atherogenic lipoproteins; also, heterogeneity of these particles has been described over recent years, and it is believed that the most atherogenic forms are dense, small and oxidized LDLs. All apoB-containing lipoproteins have an atherogenic effect, though a variable content of other apolipoproteins and triglycerides. Therefore, both LDLs and VLDLs and their remnants, as well as IDLs (intermediate density lipoproteins) are considered risk factors for atherosclerosis. The triad known as "atherogenic dyslipidemia" encompasses increased LDL (dense and small) concentration in plasma, increased VLDL remnants and reduced HDL concentration.

Lipoprotein (a) is considered an independent risk factor both in males and in females (16).

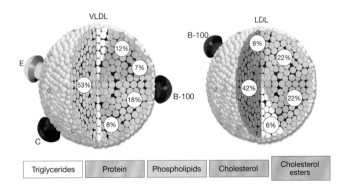

Atherogenic lipoproteins

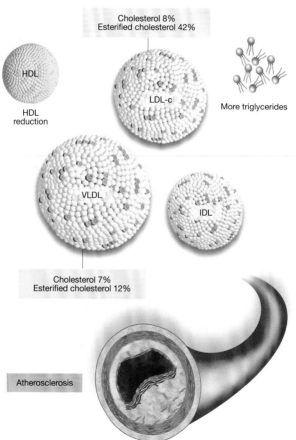

HDL

HDL
reduction

Cholesterol 8%
Esterified cholesterol 42%

LDL-c

More triglycerides

VLDL

IDL

Cholesterol 7%
Esterified cholesterol 12%

Atherosclerosis

Atherogenesis encompasses a series of highly specific cellular and molecular responses within a process of chronic inflammation. The theory supporting that this process occurs as a response to injury proposes that endothelial denudation is the first step in atherogenesis. Endothelial dysfunction may be induced by several factors (dyslipidemia, hypertension, cigarette smoking, etc.), resulting in increased endothelial permeability for lipoproteins and other plasma constituents. The initial phase of atherogenesis is characterized by a chain of events that starts with circulating monocytes "rolling" on the endothelial surface, followed by firm adhesion, activation and finally migration into the vascular wall. Once there, they can incorporate oxidized LDL (OxLDL) and become foam cells (15)(17).

Risk factors

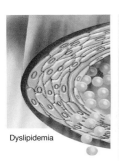 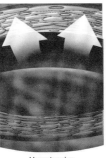

Dyslipidemia

Tobacco use (hypoxia)

Hypertension

Atherogenesis, response-to-injury hypothesis

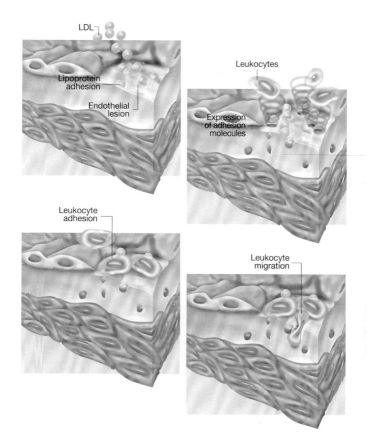

LDL

Lipoprotein adhesion

Endothelial lesion

Leukocytes

Expression of adhesion molecules

Leukocyte adhesion

Leukocyte migration

Both classical cardiovascular risk factors (dyslipidemia, hypertension, cigarette smoking, diabetes, hemorheologic factors) and others more recently involved in atherogenesis (homocysteine, free radicals, chronic viral infections and *Chlamydia*, inflammatory mechanisms and estrogen deficiency) represent chronic aggression to endothelial cells and affect their multiple functions. Prolonged exposure to these aggressive factors promotes perpetuation of the inflammatory response as well as development and complication of atherogenic lesions; this results from adhesion of plaques and monocytes to the vascular wall, infiltration by macrophages and T-cell specific subtypes, release of growth factors that induce proliferation of smooth muscle cells and abundant fibrin deposition, and disruption of thrombotic-thrombolytic equilibrium. In addition, it leads to abnormal regulation of vascular tone (18)(19).

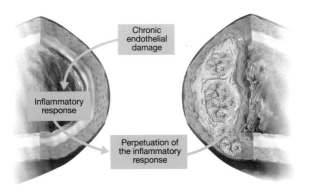

Chronic endothelial damage

Endothelial damage factors

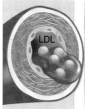

Dyslipidemia

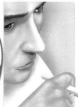

Tobacco use

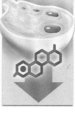

Estrogen deficit

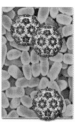

Viruses and bacteria

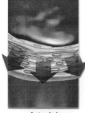

Arterial hypertension

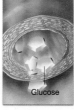

Diabetes

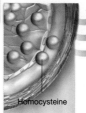

Hyperhomocysteinemia

Generation of free radicals

Endothelial dysfunction (ED) represents loss of endothelial ability to modulate vascular tone and processes such as platelet aggregation and thrombogenesis, neutrophil adhesion and cell proliferation; therefore, ED plays a significant part not only in formation of the atheromatous plaque but also in rapid progression of atherosclerosis development.

ED has been sometimes referred to as loss of endothelium-dependent vascular relaxation as a result of reduced NO bioactivity in the vascular wall. It has been shown that an impairment of endothelium-dependent vasorelaxation in coronary circulation is a prognostic factor of atherosclerosis progression as it predicts adverse cardiovascular events (18)(19).

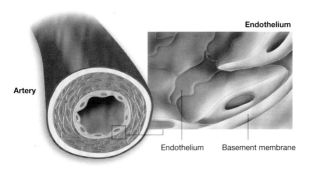

Artery

Endothelium

Endothelium   Basement membrane

Endothelial dysfunction

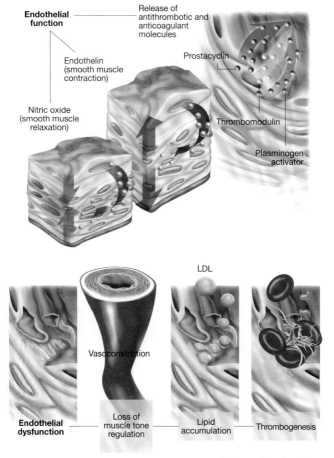

Endothelial function

Release of antithrombotic and anticoagulant molecules

Endothelin (smooth muscle contraction)

Nitric oxide (smooth muscle relaxation)

Prostacyclin

Thrombomodulin

Plasminogen activator

LDL

Vasoconstriction

Endothelial dysfunction

Loss of muscle tone regulation

Lipid accumulation

Thrombogenesis

Some of the smooth muscle cells occurring in atheromatous lesions are resident intimal cells whereas others proliferate and migrate towards the intima in response to different stimuli. These stimuli include lipid accumulation, damage to intimal cells and extracellular matrix, and deposits of platelets and fibrinogen, all of which activates resident cells to produce chemotactic and mitogenic factors. Activated endothelial cells, macrophages and other cells of the inflammatory process release growth factors: platelet derived growth factors (PDGF), fibroblast growth factors (FGF-β), and transforming growth factors (TGF-β). These induce migration and proliferation of adjacent smooth muscle cells which become intermixed with the inflammation area to form an "intermediate lesion". Muscle cells in these arterial lesions are known as "activated or metabolically active muscle cells" (15)(20).

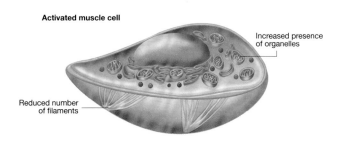

Activated muscle cell

Increased presence of organelles

Reduced number of filaments

Proliferation and migration of smooth muscle cells

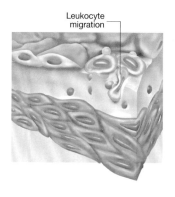

Leukocyte migration

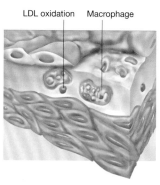

LDL oxidation

Macrophage

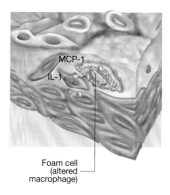

MCP-1

IL-1

Foam cell (altered macrophage)

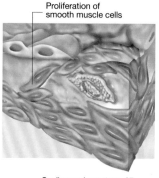

Proliferation of smooth muscle cells

MCP-1: Monocyte chemotactic protein 1

Fatty streaks are the initial lesions; they are found during the first decades of life (especially in vascular areas with nonlaminar flow and high shear stress) when an adaptive intimal thickening takes place.

Fatty streaks consist of lipid-laden monocytes and macrophages (foam cells), and T-cells, which are later joined by smooth muscle cells. Fatty streak formation includes the following steps: phagocytosis of oxidized LDL with foam cell formation (mediated by granulocyte-macrophage colony stimulating factor, interleukin-1, tumor necrosis factor α); migration and proliferation of smooth muscle cells; T-cell activation (mediated by TNF-α, interleukin-2, and granulocytemacrophage colony-stimulating factor); and platelet adhesion and migration (promoted by integrins, P-selectin, thromboxane A2, tissue factor, interleukin-8 and platelet derived factor) (15)(20).

Fatty streaks

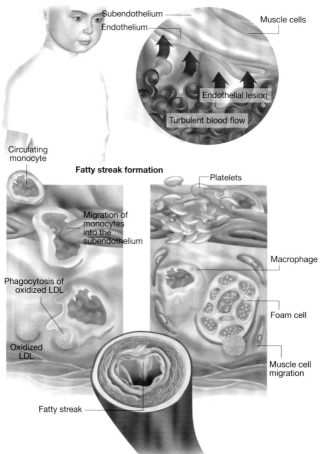

Subendothelium

Endothelium

Muscle cells

Endothelial lesion

Turbulent blood flow

Circulating monocyte

Fatty streak formation

Platelets

Migration of monocytes into the subendothelium

Macrophage

Phagocytosis of oxidized LDL

Foam cell

Oxidized LDL

Muscle cell migration

Fatty streak

Fatty streaks progress into intermediate and advanced lesions, in which a fibrotic cover or fibrous cap covers a lipid core: the fibrous plaque or atheroma. It appears in young people, initially in the same locations as adaptive intimal thickenings of the eccentric type. A dense and well-defined accumulation of extracellular lipid causes intimal disorganization, with dispersed smooth muscle cells and extracellular matrix. This lipid accumulation is referred to as lipid core. This core develops from the confluence of small isolated pools of extracellular lipid, presumed to result from continued insudation from the plasma. Between the endothelial surface and the lipid core, the proteoglycan-rich layer of the intima presents foam cells, macrophages, lymphocytes and mast cells. When connective tissue begins to form in this region, the fibrous cap may cause the lesion to be more prominent than accumulated lipid itself. It contains abundant collagen and RER-rich smooth muscle cells. The fibrous plaque obstructs the arterial lumen partially or totally, and "instability" may result in the event of fissures, hematoma or superimposed thrombus (15)(20).

Fibrous plaque formation

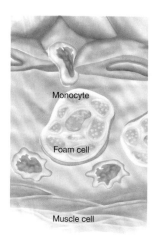

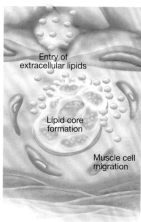

Monocyte

Foam cell

Muscle cell

Entry of extracellular lipids

Lipid core formation

Muscle cell migration

Complication - Plaque rupture

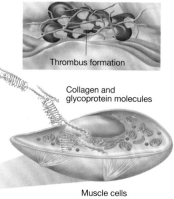

Thrombus formation

Collagen and glycoprotein molecules

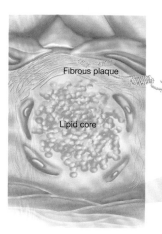

Fibrous plaque

Lipid core

Muscle cells

Atherosclerosis is a progressive disease that usually appears during the first decades of life and advances until becoming clinically evident in middle aged adults. Throughout the years, lesions go through several stages. From endothelial damage with foam cell formation they develop into fatty streaks, then they grow by accumulation of confluent lipid until the core of the atheroma and fibrous cap are established converting them into fibrous plaques. The characteristics and distribution of the lipid core and fibrous tissue as well as wall remodeling (whether eccentric or concentric) will determine the degree of vascular lumen occlusion and whether the plaque is stable or at risk for rupture, thrombosis and clinical sequelae. Plaques with a greater lipid content, a thin fibrous cap and increased leukocyte activity at the "shoulders" of the lesion are the so-called "vulnerable" plaques; they are at risk for disruption and make up what is known as acute coronary syndrome. In general, before plaque rupture these lesions only cause moderate luminal obstruction (21).

Phases in the development and expansion of a coronary atheromatous plaque

Age (in years)

10   25-35   55-65

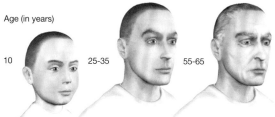

Degrees of arterial obstruction

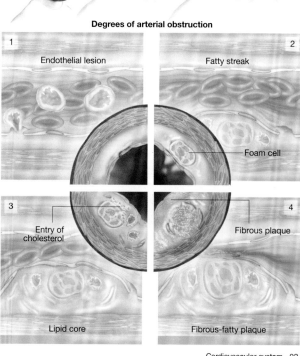

1 Endothelial lesion

2 Fatty streak

Foam cell

3 Entry of cholesterol

Lipid core

4 Fibrous plaque

Fibrous-fatty plaque

Following Herbert Stary's criteria, the American Heart Association provides a histological classification of atherosclerotic lesions. "Initial" and "intermediate" lesions are subclassified as types I, II and III. "Advanced" lesions, i.e. when accumulation of lipid, cells and matrix components are associated with structural disorganization, repair, intimal thickening and deformity of the arterial wall, are classified as types IV, V, and VI. Although generally these lesions do not narrow the arterial lumen, they may become "unstable" abruptly.

Initial lesion (type I): isolated macrophages, foam cells, adaptive thickening.

Type II lesion: "fatty streak".

Type III lesion: "preatheroma", extracellular lipid droplets disrupt the coherence of intimal smooth muscle cells. These lipids then converge in areas of dense accumulation and originate a *type IV lesion* or atheroma, with a well-defined lipid core that causes intimal disorganization. Formation of thick layers of connective tissue gives rise to a *type V lesion* or fibrous plaque (Vb or type VII lesion when calcified, and Vc or type VIII lesion if predominantly fibrous).

Type VI lesion: lesions complicated due to fissure, hematoma and/or thrombus (20).

Classification of atherosclerotic lesions

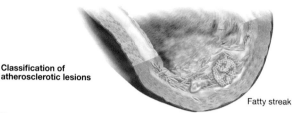

Classification of atherosclerotic lesions

Fatty streak

Type I - Initial lesion

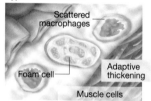

Scattered macrophages

Foam cell

Adaptive thickening

Muscle cells

Type II - Fatty streak

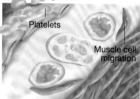

Platelets

Muscle cell migration

Type III - Preatheroma

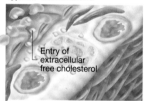

Entry of extracellular free cholesterol

Type IV - Atheroma

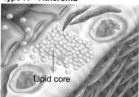

Lipid core

Type V - Fibroadipose plaque

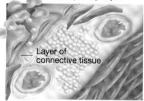

Layer of connective tissue

Type VI - Complicated lesion

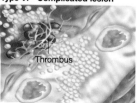

Thrombus

Atherosclerosis and its consequences

The relation between lipid content and the fibrous cap is thought to play an essential role in the natural evolution of the atheromatous plaque. It has been observed that in those atherosclerotic lesions showing a thin fibrous cap and lipid-rich content, plaques are more susceptible to complications such as rupture; for this reason, they are referred to as unstable and are prone to thrombogenesis. This resulting thrombus, together with local vasoconstriction, causes blood flow interruption leading to an imbalance between oxygen supply and demand. The arterial intima frequently presents lesions in the atheromatous plaque that promote thrombus formation.

In the early stages of plaque progression, when the plaque is not too big, it does not compromise the arterial lumen or modify the preexistent degree of ischemia. Thus, the thrombus lodges and the plaque grows without this leading to a well-defined clinical condition. However, if the vessel lumen is initially reduced, a thrombus may affect balance, trigger ischemia and consequently, worsen the clinical picture (3)(5).

Atherosclerosis, thrombosis and thromboembolism

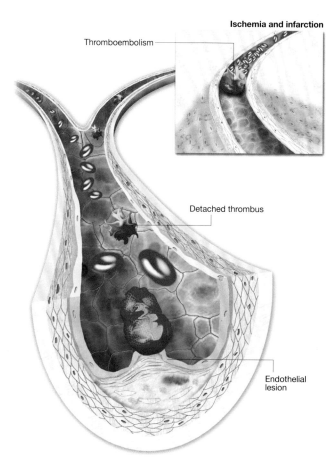

Thromboembolism

Ischemia and infarction

Detached thrombus

Endothelial lesion

Although atherosclerosis tends to occur in elastic and large arteries, distribution is not uniform. The aorta is usually severely affected, especially the abdominal aorta which is generally much more involved than the thoracic aorta. The large caliber of this artery makes it a rare site for the occurrence of occlusive symptoms although it can be the source of emboli or plaque material to peripheral branches.

After the abdominal aorta, the next most affected vessels are the coronary arteries, the lower limb arteries and the descending thoracic aorta, the internal carotid arteries and the circle of Willis vessels. Atheromas appear most frequently in the first 6 cm of the coronary tree, although they also occur in peripheral areas. Lesions are observed in the extramural portions of the coronary arteries and not in the intramural segments surrounded by muscle. Upper limb vessels are usually undamaged, as well as mesenteric and renal arteries, except at their origin (3)(5).

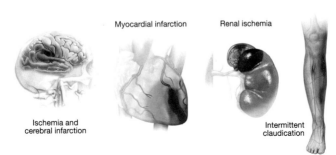

Myocardial infarction

Renal ischemia

Ischemia and
cerebral infarction

Intermittent
claudication

Main vessels affected by atherosclerosis

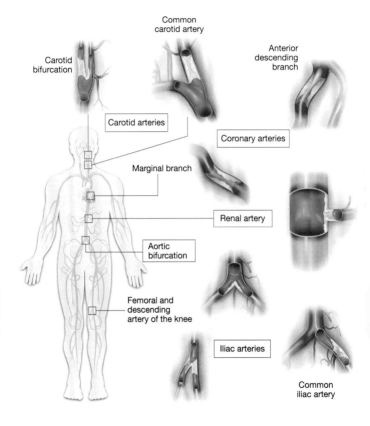

Common carotid artery

Anterior descending branch

Carotid bifurcation

Carotid arteries

Coronary arteries

Marginal branch

Renal artery

Aortic bifurcation

Femoral and descending artery of the knee

Iliac arteries

Common iliac artery

The term *ischemic heart disease* (IHD) is frequently used as a synonym for coronary heart disease (CHD) since heart ischemia in most cases results from obstruction of the coronary vessels by atherosclerotic plaques. When an atheromatous lesion produces >50% diameter stenosis, blood flow reduction leads to muscle hypoxia and late metabolite removal. The same occurs when thrombus formation follows plaque rupture.

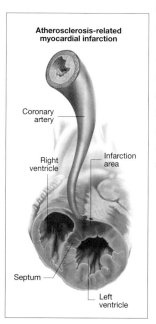

Atherosclerosis-related myocardial infarction

Coronary artery

Right ventricle

Infarction area

Septum

Left ventricle

Coronary vasospasm (dynamic obstruction of the artery) may also lead to heart ischemia as a result of inadequate perfusion.
In about 30% of patients, dysfunction of small coronary arteries and arterioles is accompanied with ischemic signs and symptoms altogether known as "microvascular angina" (22).

Ischemic heart disease

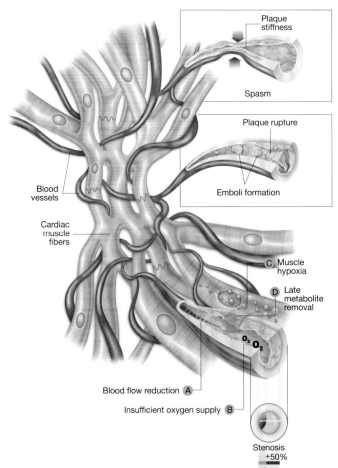

Plaque stiffness

Spasm

Plaque rupture

Emboli formation

Blood vessels

Cardiac muscle fibers

C Muscle hypoxia

D Late metabolite removal

O₂ O₂

Blood flow reduction A

Insufficient oxygen supply B

Stenosis +50%

Chronic stable angina is the most frequent anginal syndrome. It typically manifests with pain, tightness or a burning sensation in the precordial, substernal or epigastric region, with radiation to the jaw, neck or left arm. Pain usually lasts for a few minutes, very rarely between 20 and 30 minutes and is relieved by rest and sublingual nitroglycerin. Symptoms are precipitated by exertion of different degrees of intensity (physical activity, sexual intercourse, emotional stress, exposure to cold, excessive eating, smoking), but frequency and severity of symptoms do not vary and the "anginal threshold" (limitation of coronary reserve) is usually stable in each patient. The underlying cause of stable angina is fixed coronary artery stenosis that obstructs blood flow (at least 50% of the lumen). These fibrous plaques grow slowly and eventually allow for development of collateral circulation (22)(23).

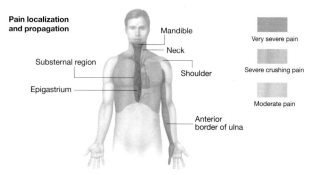

Pain localization and propagation

Mandible

Neck

Substernal region

Shoulder

Epigastrium

Anterior border of ulna

Very severe pain

Severe crushing pain

Moderate pain

Stable angina pectoris

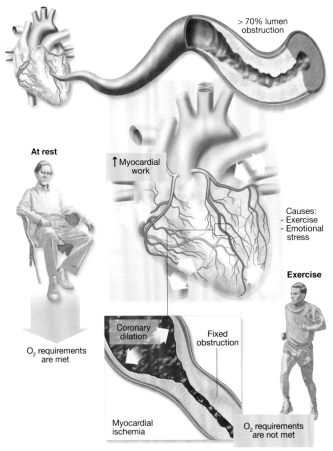

> 70% lumen obstruction

At rest

↑ Myocardial work

Causes:
- Exercise
- Emotional stress

Exercise

O₂ requirements are met

Coronary dilation

Fixed obstruction

Myocardial ischemia

O₂ requirements are not met

Unstable angina pectoris

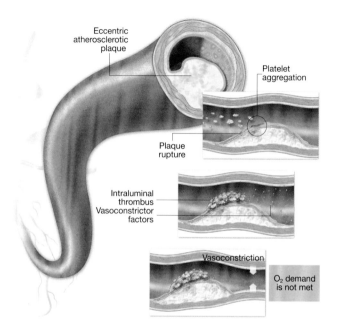

Eccentric atherosclerotic plaque

Platelet aggregation

Plaque rupture

Intraluminal thrombus
Vasoconstrictor factors

Vasoconstriction

O_2 demand is not met

Unstable angina falls within the so-called "acute coronary syndromes". It usually presents with three patterns: recent onset angina (less than 1 month), precipitated by minimal exertion; stable angina with an "in crescendo" or progressive pattern; and angina at rest. The most common physiopathological mechanism is formation of a thrombus that produces subtotal occlusion by superimposing over a fissured or eroded coronary atheromatous plaque (22)(24).

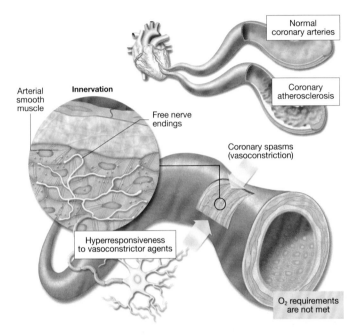

Normal coronary arteries

Coronary atherosclerosis

Arterial smooth muscle

Innervation

Free nerve endings

Coronary spasms (vasoconstriction)

Hyperresponsiveness to vasoconstrictor agents

O_2 requirements are not met

Prinzmetal angina results from transmural myocardial ischemia caused by coronary vasospasm and may occur in patients with or without coronary artery atherosclerosis; many of them have established coronary lesions but others present angiographically normal coronary arteries. Pain usually appears while at rest with no triggering factor; it generally follows a circadian pattern and is more common early in the morning (22)(24).

Clinical manifestations of chronic ischemic heart disease include asymptomatic ischemia, chronic stable angina, unstable angina, arrhythmias, myocardial infarction, chronic heart failure and death. This is the most common progression sequence throughout the years, although it may vary and even show up first with sudden death.

Currently available epidemiological studies and sophisticated diagnostic methods have revealed that a significant proportion of patients may present with chronic ischemic heart disease associated with extensive coronary atherosclerosis and still present no clinical symptoms at all. This silent ischemia is typical in diabetes (as a result of cardiac denervation in autonomic neuropathy) (22)(24).

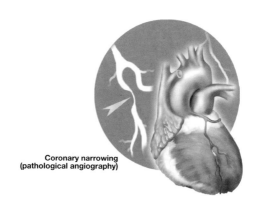

**Coronary narrowing
(pathological angiography)**

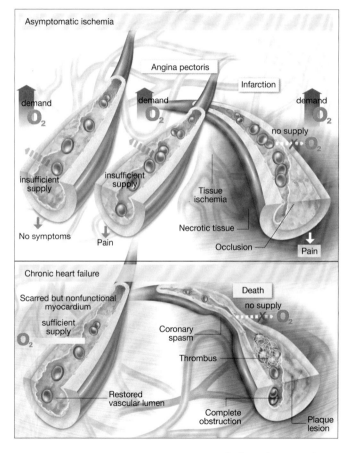

Asymptomatic ischemia

Angina pectoris

Infarction

demand O₂

demand O₂

demand O₂

no supply O₂

insufficient supply

insufficient supply

Tissue ischemia

Necrotic tissue

Occlusion

No symptoms

Pain

Pain

Chronic heart failure

Death

Scarred but nonfunctional myocardium

no supply O₂

sufficient supply

O₂

Coronary spasm

Thrombus

Restored vascular lumen

Complete obstruction

Plaque lesion

The expression myocardial infarction (MI) refers to necrosis of a group of cardiac smooth muscle cells as a result of ischemia. Coronary occlusion (either gradual or sudden) caused by progression of an atheromatous plaque is the leading cause of this event. Typical presentation includes severe and long-lasting chest or epigastric pain, radiating to the left upper arm and the jaw; it can be accompanied with dyspnea, sweating, nausea or vomiting. According to the wall involved, MIs can be classified as transmural, subendocardial or intramural. According to location, they can be anterior, posterior, diaphragmatic, septal or combined (the latter being the most frequent ones); all of these involve some area of the left ventricle (Vl). Purely atrial or right ventricle (RV) infarctions are rare; however, RV involvement is common as an extension of a LV posteroseptal MI. These locations are related to the coronary artery involved by occlusion (25).

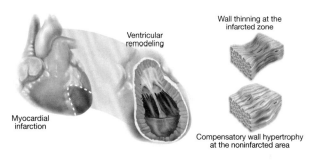

Ventricular remodeling

Wall thinning at the infarcted zone

Myocardial infarction

Compensatory wall hypertrophy at the noninfarcted area

Myocardial infarction

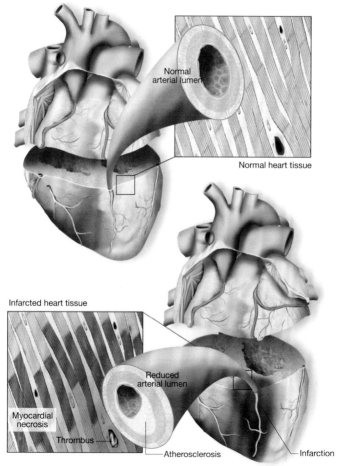

Normal arterial lumen

Normal heart tissue

Infarcted heart tissue

Reduced arterial lumen

Myocardial necrosis

Thrombus

Atherosclerosis

Infarction

Initial lesions of myocardial necrosis secondary to ischemia are produced in the subendocardial region and later extend to the epicardium; if coronary obstruction is total and sustained after 4 hours of interrupted blood flow, 70-90% of the myocardium distal to the lesion shows ischemia and then necrosis.

Infarction is confined to the subendocardial region when coronary obstruction is incomplete or there is significant collateral circulation (also, when the artery involved is revascularized by thrombolysis or angioplasty within the first hours of the event). In transmural infarction, the lesion involves the wall from the endocardium to the epicardium. This kind of transmural MI has traditionally been considered to present a Q wave pattern on ECG whereas subendocardial MI is associated with changes in the ST-T segment only without Q wave. Currently, the most common names are NQMI (non Q wave myocardial infarction) instead of subendocardial infarction, and QwMI (Q wave myocardial infarction) instead of transmural infarction (25)(26)(27).

Subendocardial vs. transmural infarction

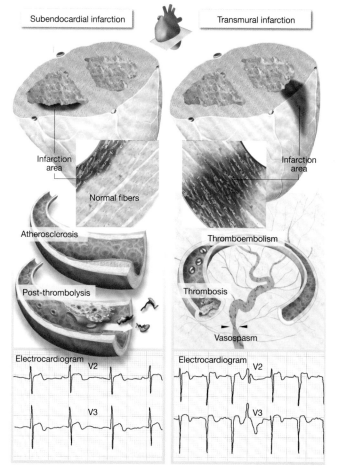

Subendocardial infarction

Transmural infarction

Infarction area

Normal fibers

Infarction area

Atherosclerosis

Thromboembolism

Post-thrombolysis

Thrombosis

Vasospasm

Electrocardiogram   V2

Electrocardiogram   V2

V3

V3

Necrosis is microscopically recognized after 6-8 hours of development; however, macroscopic detection takes 18-24 hours after ischemia is established. It first shows as a pale grayish ill-defined territory, and during the following days it becomes a brownish-yellow swollen area with map-like, hyperemic rims. Leukocyte infiltration occurs and peaks on the 4th. or 5th. day, followed by macrophages, hemosiderin and newly formed blood vessels; also, endocardial fibroelastosis develops. During the second week, when fatty change occurs, the infarcted area shows an intense yellow color, becomes friable and slightly depressed. In this –resorptive– stage, myocardial fiber detritus is found in the cytoplasm of macrophages as well as infiltration of granulation tissue. Collagen-producing myofibroblasts are observed in granulation tissue. Towards the third week, the infarcted territory is soft, somewhat elastic, and reddish due to engorgement of newly formed vessels; also, it presents lymphoplasmacytic infiltrate. From the fourth week onwards it becomes firmer and grayish, and gradually retracts due to scarring; collagen is abundant and dense. In general, scarring is very advanced by the sixth week although complete replacement depends on the infarction size (26)(28).

Morphologic progression of myocardial damage

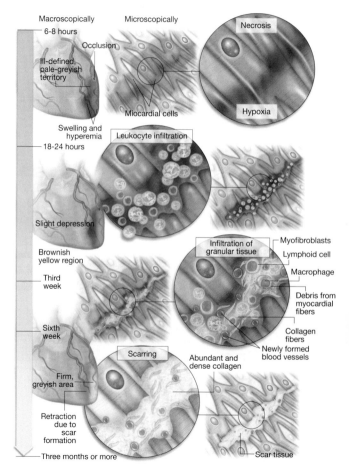

Macroscopically

6-8 hours

Occlusion

Ill-defined, pale-greyish territory

Microscopically

Miocardial cells

Necrosis

Hypoxia

Swelling and hyperemia

18-24 hours

Slight depression

Leukocyte infiltration

Brownish yellow region

Third week

Sixth week

Infiltration of granular tissue

Myofibroblasts

Lymphoid cell

Macrophage

Debris from myocardial fibers

Collagen fibers

Newly formed blood vessels

Firm, greyish area

Retraction due to scar formation

Scarring

Abundant and dense collagen

Scar tissue

Three months or more

An electrocardiogram (ECG) may show signs of myocardial ischemia, in particular changes in the ST segment and the T wave, and necrosis signs, such as changes of the QRS complex.

In the absence of electrocardiographic standards that might lead to confusion (such as right branch blockage, left ventricular hypertrophy, etc.) the following criteria have been adopted for the electrocardiographic diagnosis of ischemia: -in patients with an ST segment elevation: new or allegedly new ST segment elevation in point J in two o more adjoining leads with cut-off points over 0.2 mV in leads V1, V2, or V3, and over or equal to 0.1 mV in other leads. -In patients without an ST segment elevation: depression of ST or only T wave abnormalities.

They must be present in two or more adjoining leads, and at least in two ECG recordings taken several hours apart.

Changes commonly observed in an established infarction are: any Q wave in leads V1 to V3; Q wave 30 ms or more in leads I, II, aVL, aVF, V4, V5, V6. Changes in Q wave must be 1 mm deep or more and occur in two adjoining leads (27)(29).

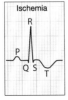 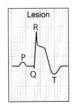 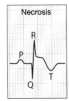

Electrocardiogram and myocardial infarction

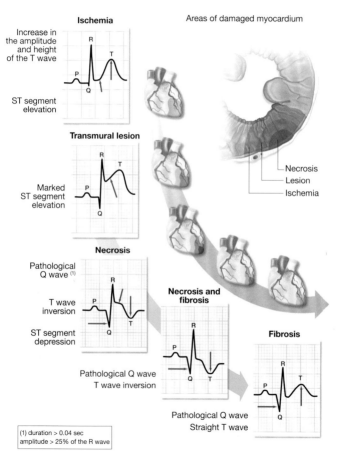

Ischemia

Increase in the amplitude and height of the T wave

ST segment elevation

Transmural lesion

Marked ST segment elevation

Necrosis

Pathological Q wave (1)

T wave inversion

ST segment depression

Necrosis and fibrosis

Pathological Q wave
T wave inversion

Fibrosis

Pathological Q wave
Straight T wave

Areas of damaged myocardium

Necrosis
Lesion
Ischemia

(1) duration > 0.04 sec
amplitude > 25% of the R wave

Complications of infarction, cardiogenic shock

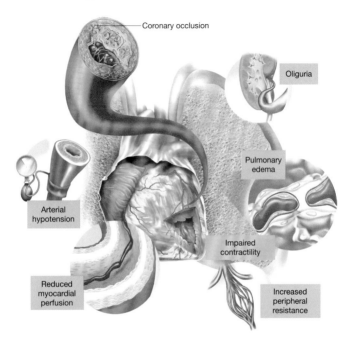

Coronary occlusion

Oliguria

Pulmonary edema

Arterial hypotension

Impaired contractility

Reduced myocardial perfusion

Increased peripheral resistance

Cardiogenic shock is the most serious complication of acute myocardial infarction (AMI) and has an ominous prognosis: in-hospital mortality is between 70 and 100%. This complication results from severe ventricular dysfunction, which may be a consequence of extensive AMI or less severe necrosis, but in patients with an already impaired myocardial function or following myocardial rupture (30).

Infarction complications, arrhythmias

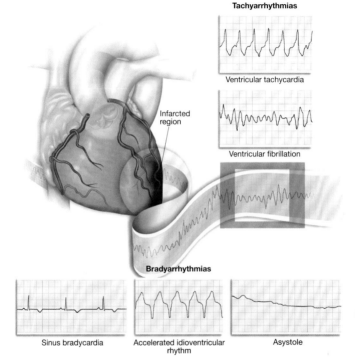

Tachyarrhythmias

Ventricular tachycardia

Ventricular fibrillation

Infarcted region

Bradyarrhythmias

Sinus bradycardia

Accelerated idioventricular rhythm

Asystole

Post AMI complications may include tachyarrhythmias, bradyarrhythmias or high-degree heart block.
Arrhythmias are frequent during the acute phase of AMI, especially ventricular arrhythmias such as ventricular fibrillation and tachycardia, which are life-threatening (30).

Infarction complications, heart rupture

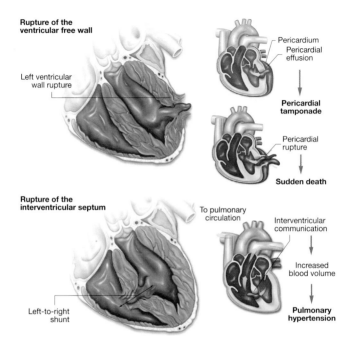

Rupture of the ventricular free wall

Left ventricular wall rupture

Pericardium
Pericardial effusion

↓

Pericardial tamponade

Pericardial rupture

↓

Sudden death

Rupture of the interventricular septum

To pulmonary circulation

Interventricular communication

↓

Increased blood volume

↓

Pulmonary hypertension

Left-to-right shunt

Among the causes for heart rupture, the most frequent is free wall rupture, 8 or 10-fold more common than that of other myocardial structures (interventricular septum or papillary muscles). Free wall rupture accounts for up to 10% of deaths from AMI; it is more common in females, people with hypertension and the elderly. It is associated with transmural infarction and may occur in both ventricles (30).

Complications of infarction, ventricular aneurysm and cardiac thrombosis

Ventricular aneurysm

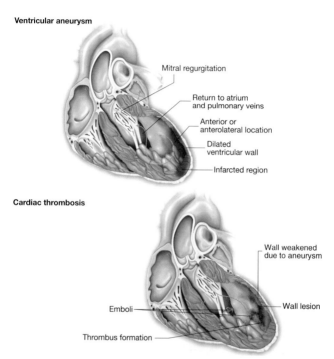

Mitral regurgitation

Return to atrium and pulmonary veins

Anterior or anterolateral location

Dilated ventricular wall

Infarcted region

Cardiac thrombosis

Wall weakened due to aneurysm

Wall lesion

Emboli

Thrombus formation

Ventricular aneurysm occurs in 12 to 15% of patients who survive an AMI. It generally affects the left ventricle in the apex and anterior wall. *Cardiac thrombosis* occurs in almost 30% of recent infarctions; the true relevance of mural thrombosis lies in its potential to cause embolism (30).

Myocardial infarction mainly affects the left ventricle; however, between 25 and 40% of infarctions involving the diaphragmatic surface compromise the right ventricle. Inferior AMI affecting the right ventricle (RV) is associated with a significantly higher mortality rate (25 to 30%) than that of patients with inferior AMI without RV involvement (6%) therefore the former should be considered high risk patients and high priority candidates for reperfusion therapy. The clinical presentation of patients with RV infarction encompasses from asymptomatic individuals with mild right ventricular dysfunction to patients with cardiogenic shock. Significant hemodynamic compromise associated with anterior infarction or isolated RV infarction is rare (30).

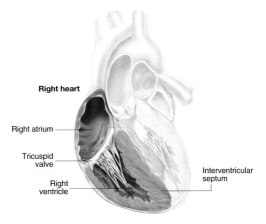

Right heart

Right atrium

Tricuspid
valve

Right
ventricle

Interventricular
septum

Right ventricular infarction

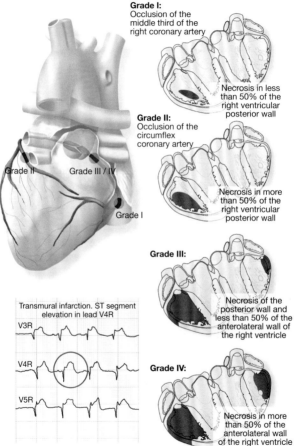

Grade I:
Occlusion of the middle third of the right coronary artery

Necrosis in less than 50% of the right ventricular posterior wall

Grade II:
Occlusion of the circumflex coronary artery

Necrosis in more than 50% of the right ventricular posterior wall

Grade II

Grade III / IV

Grade I

Grade III:
Necrosis of the posterior wall and less than 50% of the anterolateral wall of the right ventricle

Grade IV:
Necrosis in more than 50% of the anterolateral wall of the right ventricle

Transmural infarction. ST segment elevation in lead V4R

V3R

V4R

V5R

Diagnosis of acute myocardial infarction (AMI) is based on three parameters: ECG changes (present in subsequent recordings), biochemical markers of myocardial injury, and clinical symptoms. Diagnostic confirmation of AMI depends on the presence of two of the three mentioned criteria. Clinical symptoms of ischemia include: chest pain and sensation of imminent death (angor animi); intense chest discomfort, tightness or pressure, which may radiate to the epigastrium, jaw, left arm, and back. Chest pain lasts about 30 minutes and appears both during exertion and at rest. AMI is usually associated with dyspnea, diaphoresis, nausea and vomiting, dizziness and syncope. Although this is the typical picture, patients with AMI may refer only epigastric pain or may even develop a silent MI, which may be diagnosed by ECG, laboratory tests or diagnostic imaging. In the elderly, certain symptoms such as dyspnea, dizziness, or symptoms of cardiovascular arrhythmia may dominate the clinical presentation (25)(30).

Diagnostic triad of AMI

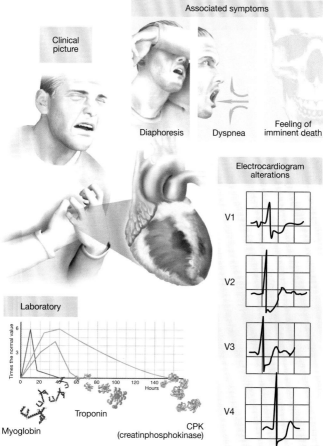

Clinical picture

Associated symptoms

Diaphoresis

Dyspnea

Feeling of imminent death

Electrocardiogram alterations

V1

V2

V3

V4

Laboratory

Times the normal value

Hours

Myoglobin

Troponin

CPK (creatinphosphokinase)

The common carotid artery (CCA) and its two branches (external and internal) supply the skull and brain and, together with the vertebral artery system, form the cerebral circulation circuit. Internal carotid arteries are a common site of atherosclerosis. In the internal carotid arteries atheromatous plaques are characterized by being particularly fragile, ulcerated, with superimposed thrombosis. Apparently, atheromatous plaques in these arteries present a thinner fibrous layer which facilitates ulceration, rupture and secondary thrombosis.

A carotid bruit detected on systematic physical examination is a sign of atheromatosis. When stenosis is greater, clinical signs may appear such as amaurosis fugax or disorders related to sensitivity or muscle strength in the limbs or the face on the opposite side of the artery involved (31)(32).

Most frequent locations

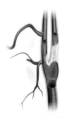 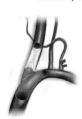 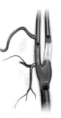 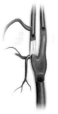

| Carotid bifurcation | Common carotid artery | Internal carotid artery | External carotid artery |

Carotid atherosclerosis

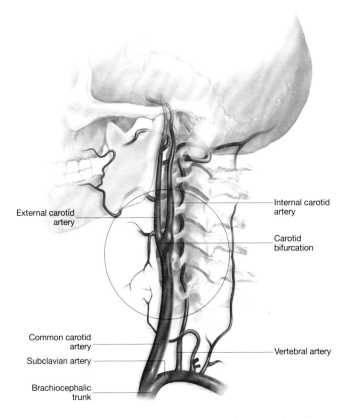

External carotid artery

Internal carotid artery

Carotid bifurcation

Common carotid artery

Subclavian artery

Brachiocephalic trunk

Vertebral artery

The clinical presentation of ischemic stroke is characterized by sudden onset of focal neurological symptoms as a result of an affected vascular territory, which provide an indication of the location and identification of the vessel and anatomical pathology. For example, lesions located at the lateral aspect of the cerebral hemisphere (territory of the middle cerebral artery) will present with the following signs and symptoms: hemiparesis, hemihypesthesia, motor aphasia, central aphasia, apraxia and hemianopia. If located in the midbrain (territory of the posterior cerebral artery) they will cause ipsilateral paralysis of the third cranial nerve and contralateral hemiplegia. If the medulla oblongata is affected (vertebral and posterior inferior cerebellar artery), they will be accompanied by hemiplegia sparing the face and altered contralateral proprioceptive sensitivity, ipsilateral hypoglossal paralysis and a lateral syndrome that includes hypesthesia, nystagmus, ataxia and ipsilateral paralysis of the 9th., 10th. and 11th. cranial nerves, with contralateral thermalgesia (32)(33).

Clinical consequences of ischemic stroke

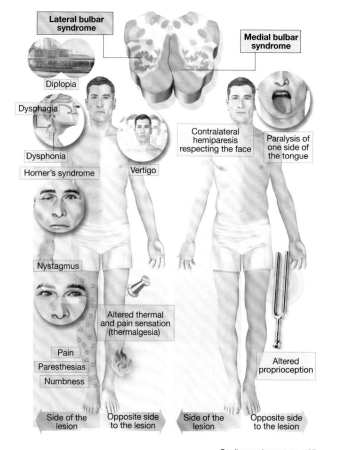

Lateral bulbar syndrome

Medial bulbar syndrome

Diplopia

Dysphagia

Dysphonia

Horner's syndrome

Vertigo

Contralateral hemiparesis respecting the face

Paralysis of one side of the tongue

Nystagmus

Altered thermal and pain sensation (thermalgesia)

Pain

Paresthesias

Numbness

Altered proprioception

Side of the lesion

Opposite side to the lesion

Side of the lesion

Opposite side to the lesion

Occlusion of the superficial femoral artery is the most common form of peripheral occlusive vascular disease. The terminal aorta and the iliac and popliteal arteries are next in frequency. The time the blockage takes to develop, as well as its location and magnitude, will determine the symptoms. Onset of ischemia may be gradual or acute. Sudden and complete occlusion of the terminal segment of the aorta or its iliac branches may result from a lodged embolus, superimposed thrombosis following a plaque rupture or an aneurysm rupture. In this case, onset of clinical manifestations is sudden and dramatic, and usually characterized by a very severe pain in the non-irrigated area.

Progressive ischemia (related to atheromatous plaque growth) will cause pain in the gluteal muscles and in the lower limbs upon walking, absence of femoral pulse and, very often, a murmur in the femoral artery. In men, sexual impotence is an additional finding (13)(34).

Most frequent locations

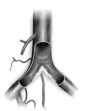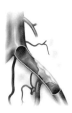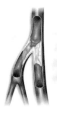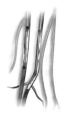

| Aortic bifurcation | Common iliac artery | Femoral and descending artery of the knee | Dorsal artery of the foot and peroneal artery |

Iliac artery atherosclerosis

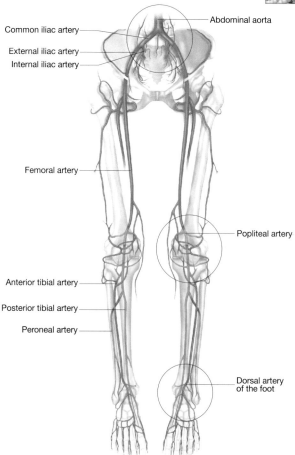

Abdominal aorta

Common iliac artery

External iliac artery

Internal iliac artery

Femoral artery

Popliteal artery

Anterior tibial artery

Posterior tibial artery

Peroneal artery

Dorsal artery of the foot

The typical symptom indicating arterial atherosclerotic involvement in the lower limbs is intermittent claudication: muscular, cramp-like pain in the lower limbs upon walking which disappears by resting, together with absent or weak pulses. The calves are the most frequently affected site, but the condition may involve other regions which are evidenced by the topography of the obstructive lesion: femoropopliteal region, in the calves; aortoiliac, in the gluteal region; popliteal and tibiofibular, in the ankle and foot.

In the most advanced stages this pain is constant, ultimately affecting underlying tissues. The severity of claudication symptoms is proportional to the degree of arterial involvement and the degree of ischemia in the irrigated region; pain upon walking can progress to pain at rest. Under these critical conditions of limb ischemia, ulcers, necrosis and gangrene may occur as a result of even minimal trauma (13)(34).

Intermittent claudication

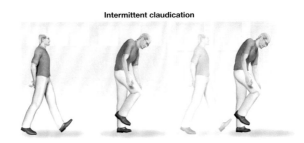

Intermittent claudication

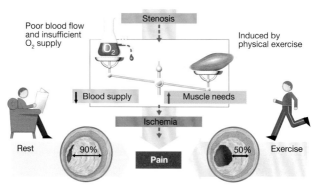

Stenosis

Poor blood flow
and insufficient
O_2 supply

O_2

Induced by
physical exercise

↓ Blood supply | ↑ Muscle needs

Ischemia

Pain

Rest — 90%

50% — Exercise

Clinical characteristics

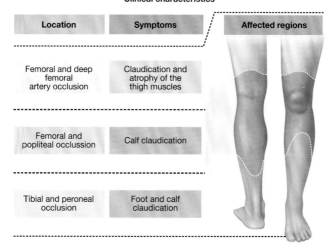

Location	Symptoms	Affected regions
Femoral and deep femoral artery occlusion	Claudication and atrophy of the thigh muscles	
Femoral and popliteal occlusion	Calf claudication	
Tibial and peroneal occlusion	Foot and calf claudication	

It is estimated that in at least 5 to 15% of the annual new cases of dialysis due to renal failure, atherosclerotic renovascular disease is the major cause.

This location becomes more and more frequent as the elderly population increases. It typically occurs in men over 50 years of age, smokers, with generalized atherosclerotic involvement. Patients usually present with hypertension and different degrees of renal failure; however, it may also be a silent condition detected upon necropsy. Atheromatous plaques may be found in vessels of different caliber, although they are usually located in the ostium of the renal artery. Multiple lesions may exist, and ulcerated atheromatous plaques may also generate cholesterol microemboli. These can lodge in the small peripheral arteries (arcuate, interlobular, renal, terminal or glomeruli) (35)(36).

Most frequent locations

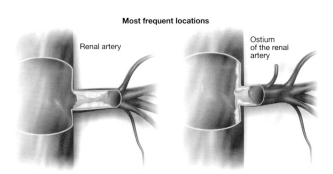

Renal artery

Ostium of the renal artery

Renal atherosclerosis

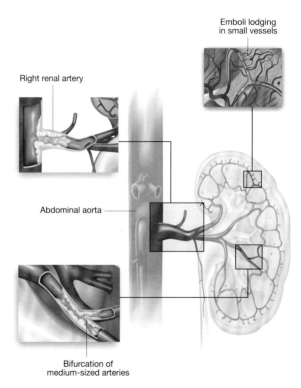

Emboli lodging
in small vessels

Right renal artery

Abdominal aorta

Bifurcation of
medium-sized arteries

Renovascular hypertension associated with unilateral or bilateral atherosclerotic narrowing of the renal arteries is present in more than one third of the patients with malignant or drug-resistant hypertension. It is the most frequent cause of secondary hypertension and usually involves a reduction in the renal artery diameter secondary to atherosclerosis. Stenosis of the renal arteries reduces blood supply to the kidney and stimulates the release and activation of the renin-angiotensin-aldosterone system. Peripheral resistance is increased, as well as water and sodium reabsorption with the corresponding expansion in plasma volume. When only one kidney is affected, the excessive increase in plasma renin activity may go unnoticed since the healthy kidney compensates by decreasing renin release. Renovascular hypertension is accompanied by grade III or IV hypertensive retinopathy, and a midepigastric systolic/diastolic murmur may be auscultated (35)(36).

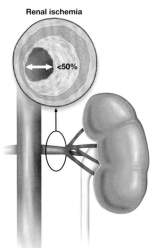

Renal ischemia

<50%

Renovascular hypertension

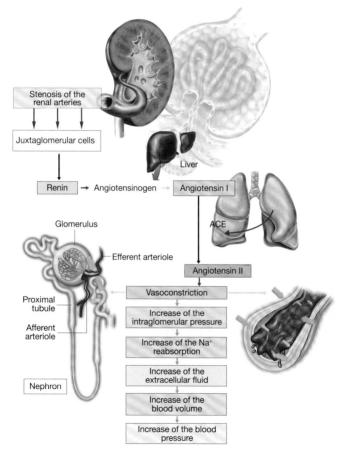

Stenosis of the
renal arteries

Juxtaglomerular cells

Renin → Angiotensinogen → Angiotensin I

Liver

ACE

Angiotensin II

Glomerulus

Efferent arteriole

Proximal
tubule

Afferent
arteriole

Nephron

Vasoconstriction

Increase of the
intraglomerular pressure

Increase of the Na$^+$
reabsorption

Increase of the
extracellular fluid

Increase of the
blood volume

Increase of the blood
pressure

Heart failure

The myocardium is composed of myocardial fibers, interstitial connective tissue and blood vessels. The inner structure of myocardial fibers differs from that of the skeletal striated muscle in their typical branching and central nuclei. The intercalated disk separates the individual fibers at the point where branched fibers join.

In a *normal heart*, most of the ventricular emptying strength results from inherent myocardial properties, specifically fiber length and force of contraction (inotropism). According to Frank-Starling law, the initial length of myocardial fibers determines increased contractility. In the presence of *heart failure*, myocardial fibers may suffer initial hypertrophy in response to increased chamber pressure, but they finally stretch as a result of continuous volume increase. Even with a severely impaired heart contractility, this compensation mechanism is usually capable of maintaining a normal cardiac output, at least, at rest. However, if it stretches beyond the so-called "optimal length" of the fiber, the force of contraction will decrease (2)(3)(5).

Normal and hypertrophic myocardial fibers

Myosin with normal ATPase activity

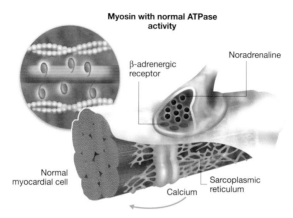

β-adrenergic receptor

Noradrenaline

Normal myocardial cell

Calcium

Sarcoplasmic reticulum

Increased myosin isoenzyme with low ATPase activity

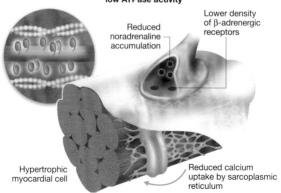

Reduced noradrenaline accumulation

Lower density of β-adrenergic receptors

Hypertrophic myocardial cell

Reduced calcium uptake by sarcoplasmic reticulum

Although the heart is a single organ, it can be functionally divided into left heart –left cavity– and right heart –right cavity.

Similarly, heart failure can be classified as right heart failure when the right ventricle is affected, and left heart failure when the left ventricle is affected.

Most clinical manifestations of heart failure are a consequence of fluid accumulation behind one of the ventricles. Left heart failure is accompanied by pulmonary congestion and the resulting dyspnea; in right heart failure, venous congestion is systemic, therefore edema appears.

If either right or left heart failure persists for long, most cases progress to congestive heart failure, characterized by failure of both ventricles, although one ventricle is always more affected than the other. Congestive heart failure is frequently a consequence of ventricular failure (2)(3).

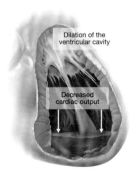

Dilation of the
ventricular cavity

Decreased
cardiac output

Types of heart failure

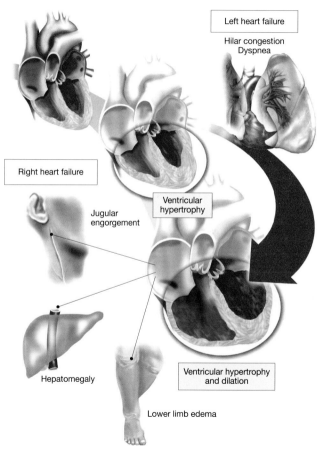

Left heart failure

Hilar congestion
Dyspnea

Right heart failure

Ventricular
hypertrophy

Jugular
engorgement

Hepatomegaly

Ventricular hypertrophy
and dilation

Lower limb edema

Left heart failure.
Predisposing factors

Over time, hypertensive heart disease can lead to heart failure. It occurs in patients with hypertension who progressively develop left ventricular hypertrophy due to long-standing chronic elevation of blood pressure. This pressure overload results from increased afterload due to the elevation of peripheral vascular resistance. Also, hypertension accelerates the development of atherosclerosis, thus reducing distensibility of the great vessels and promoting abnormal thickening of the walls of small arteries and arterioles.

Myocardial fiber hypertrophy enables the heart to overcome increased vascular resistance and maintain a normal cardiac output. Hypertrophy, in turn, increases myocardial oxygen demand and, with time, fibers become unable to contract adequately. Consequently, in the late stages of disease, myocardial dilation and congestive heart failure ensue. As it happens in some cases of renal hypertension or hypertension after stopping prolonged medication, it is also possible that a sudden and excessive elevation of blood pressure induces manifestations of a previously asymptomatic heart failure. In most cases, these presentations occur during the night while the patient is sleeping, and usually manifest as paroxysmal dyspnea (2)(3).

Hypertension

Arterial hypertension

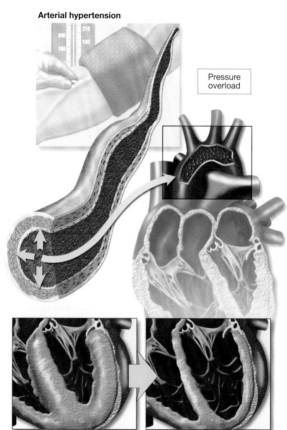

Pressure overload

Concentric hypertrophy

Ventricular dilation and failure

Progression of aortic stenosis depends on the magnitude of the defect; it can be mild, moderate or severe. Aortic stenosis symptoms, especially angina, dyspnea or exertional syncope, are markers of bad prognosis, and in the absence of treatment, death will occur within a period of 4 or 5 years. Calcification develops in almost all cases of aortic stenosis, which may worsen valve rigidity and even cause valve immobilization. Obstruction of the left ventricular outflow tract leads to a pressure gradient between the left ventricle and the aorta during systole, i.e. a pressure overload that increases gradually over the years.

The same as in hypertension, patients develop myocardial hypertrophy in order to maintain left ventricular output. Patients can exhibit increased pressure gradient for many years without a reduction in cardiac output or ventricular dilation. As stenosis becomes more severe, left ventricular systolic pressure is higher and pressure overload is increased; ultimately, progressive cardiac dilation and heart failure develop (2)(3).

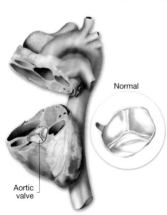

Normal

Aortic valve

Valvular heart diseases: aortic stenosis

Valve calcification and stiffness

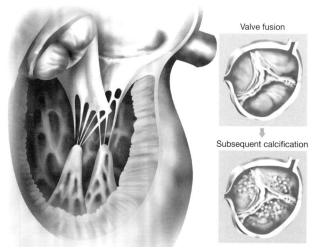

Valve fusion

Subsequent calcification

Myocardial effect

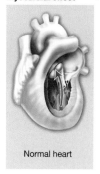

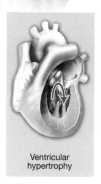

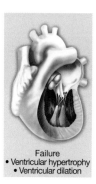

Normal heart

Ventricular hypertrophy

Failure
• Ventricular hypertrophy
• Ventricular dilation

The main hemodynamic changes related to aortic regurgitation (aka, aortic insufficiency) are left ventricular volume overload and reduced coronary artery diastolic flow. During the early stages of disease, end-diastolic left ventricular pressure is normal or appears slightly increased. As volume overload increases, end-diastolic pressure also does and there is ventricular cavity dilation. Though volume overload can be very well tolerated for many years, there is eventually a gradual reduction in myocardial inotropic state, which progressively leads to heart failure. When there is left ventricular failure in a patient with aortic regurgitation, the chances of compensation are lesser than in other types of left ventricular failure, since the ventricle is permanently subjected to an increasing volume overload. Thus, once insufficiency has developed, the prognosis is poor (2)(3).

Aortic valve failure (with diastolic regurgitation)

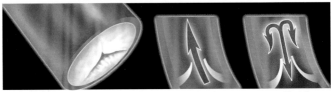

Systole   Diastole

Valvular heart diseases: aortic regurgitation

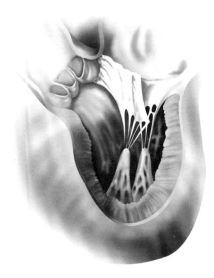

Normal aortic valve
(without diastolic
regurgitation)

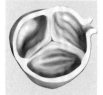

Aortic valve failure
(with diastolic
regurgitation)

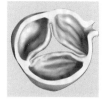

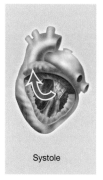

Systole

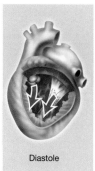

Diastole

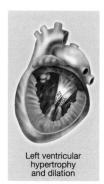

Left ventricular
hypertrophy
and dilation

Mitral regurgitation during ventricular systole allows blood to flow back to the left atrium and pulmonary veins. In chronic mitral regurgitation there is also volume overload on the left ventricle, and the volume of regurgitant blood will determine the increase in end-diastolic volume.

The left ventricle is forced to work harder and ventricular preload increases. As a result, there is an increase in the amount of blood ejected during systole and a state of elevated cardiac output. If this critical hemodynamic condition persists, the contractile properties of the left ventricular myocardium are impaired, and patients progressively develop heart failure.

The period between the occurrence of physical findings (mainly, holosystolic murmur) and the appearance of left ventricular failure symptoms varies according to the cause and degree of the insufficiency. In patients with mitral regurgitation of sudden onset

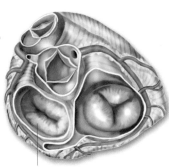

attributable to tendon rupture in the course of a myocardial infarction, left ventricular dysfunction occurs at an early stage; when mitral regurgitation is associated with rheumatic disease, a period of 20 year can elapse before the first signs of heart failure are manifested (2)(3).

Closed mitral valve

Valvular heart diseases: mitral regurgitation

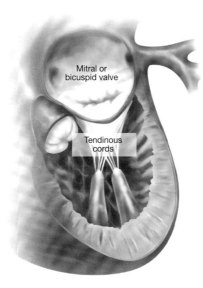

Mitral or bicuspid valve

Tendinous cords

Rupture of tendinous cords

Cusp retraction

Valve ring dilation

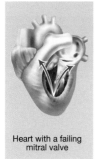

Heart with a failing mitral valve

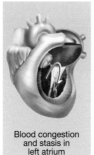

Blood congestion and stasis in left atrium

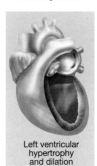

Left ventricular hypertrophy and dilation

Coarctation of the aorta is a congenital vascular disease consisting of intimal and medial proliferation with significant narrowing of the aortic lumen. This stenosis may be proximal or distal to the ductus arteriosus that during embryonic life communicates the pulmonary artery with the aorta. Constriction –of variable length– leads to an increase in blood pressure values. Blood pressure elevation occurs in the vessels that arise above the coarctation, whereas both blood pressure and pulse pressure values are lower below the narrow spot. Aortic coarctation is associated with a large collateral circulation which allows blood to "detour" around the site of narrowing. However, if it persists over time, the hypertensive state can result in progressive development of coronary heart disease, congestive heart failure or intracranial bleeding. Chronic pressure overload on the left ventricle causes a variety of events similar to those observed in patients with hypertension: –> dilation –> heart failure (2)(3).

Coarctation of the aorta

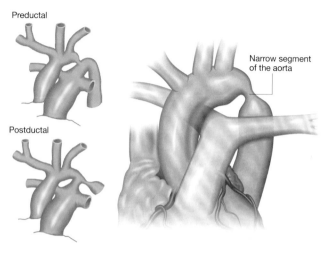

Preductal

Postductal

Narrow segment of the aorta

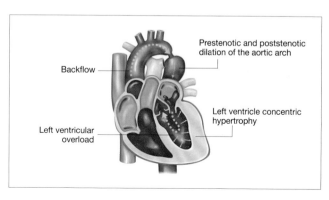

Backflow

Prestenotic and poststenotic dilation of the aortic arch

Left ventricle concentric hypertrophy

Left ventricular overload

Left heart failure.
Clinical manifestations

The main signs and symptoms of left heart failure can be observed in the lungs since there is pulmonary venous stasis (backward failure). However, there are also signs of forward failure, dependent on cardiac output decrease.

• Dyspnea: at first, it appears during exercise, and with time, it occurs even with minor efforts. It is due to increased left ventricular filling pressure which raises left atrial mean pressure and pulmonary venous and capillary pressures. Interstitial edema decreases airway compliance.

In this context, in order to achieve adequate distension, oxygen consumption is increased thus worsening dyspnea.

• Cough: dry and persistent cough, mainly at night with certain recumbent positions or during the day upon exertion. In severe failure, patients may cough up phlegm tinged with blood.

• Acute pulmonary edema: as a result of acute left ventricular failure. It causes paroxysmal nocturnal dyspnea associated with "bubbling" breath, cough with white or pink-tinged frothy sputum and basal pulmonary rales which extend rapidly. Patients have persistent orthopnea.

• The presence of tachycardia and moderately decreased systolic blood pressure indicates a reduction in cardiac output (2)(3).

Left heart failure

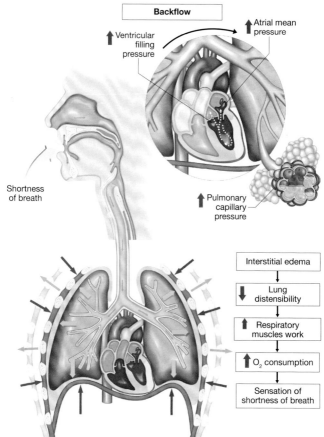

Backflow

↑ Ventricular filling pressure

↑ Atrial mean pressure

↑ Pulmonary capillary pressure

Shortness of breath

Interstitial edema

↓ Lung distensibility

↑ Respiratory muscles work

↑ O_2 consumption

Sensation of shortness of breath

In an acute episode of left ventricular failure, the inability of the myocardium to pump enough blood from the right ventricle can result in a sudden increase of pulmonary venous and capillary pressure, followed by interstitial and alveolar flooding.

The resulting pulmonary edema is a consequence of the increase in left ventricular filling pressure, which is transmitted in retrograde fashion. At this stage, the patient presents with orthopnea (shortness of breath when lying down).

When edema is limited to pulmonary interstitial spaces, the breathing rate is increased because lung stiffness causes alveolar hyperventilation and respiratory alkalosis. Conversely, when fluid leaks into the terminal bronchioles and comes up through the respiratory tree, respiratory acidosis may occur due to an alteration of the ventilation-perfusion ratio.

Early symptoms include cough, dyspnea and rales, and often a tight feeling in the chest.

As it worsens, the patient is pale, sweaty and cyanotic, breathes with difficulty, and expectorates frothy sputum, sometimes tinged with blood; rales extend upward very fast and can be heard throughout the lung fields (2)(3).

Acute pulmonary edema

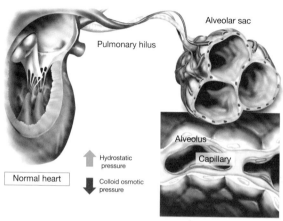

Alveolar sac

Pulmonary hilus

Alveolus

Capillary

Hydrostatic pressure

Colloid osmotic pressure

Normal heart

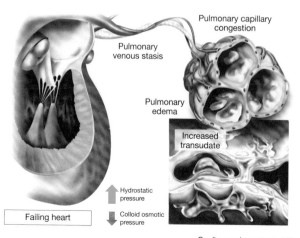

Pulmonary capillary congestion

Pulmonary venous stasis

Pulmonary edema

Increased transudate

Hydrostatic pressure

Colloid osmotic pressure

Failing heart

Right heart failure.
Predisposing factors

Pulmonary hypertension is the most common cause of
right heart failure.

Any underlying condition or disorder likely to obstruct pulmonary
circulation, either by increasing resistance or causing a sustained
increase in blood flow can lead to pulmonary hypertension.

Thus, mitral stenosis and left ventricular failure cause pulmonary
hypertension due to backward failure of the left ventricle.

Chronic pulmonary disease can lead to a reduction in the
pulmonary vascular bed as it virtually occurs in pulmonary
embolism.

When pulmonary hypertension is basically related to excessive
blood flow, the existing balance between blood flow per unit
time and pulmonary vascular resistance breaks down. This occurs
because the adaptability of the capillary bed, anatomically arranged
to allow for relatively high blood flow rates at low pressure,
is exceeded (2)(3).

Pulmonary hypertension

Pulmonary pressure > 20 mm Hg at rest

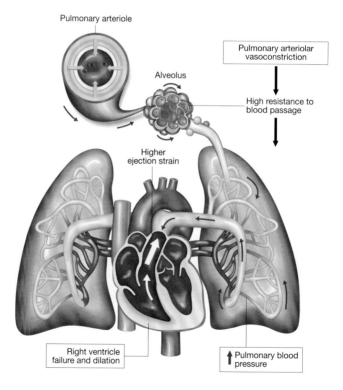

Pulmonary arteriole

Alveolus

Pulmonary arteriolar vasoconstriction

High resistance to blood passage

Higher ejection strain

Right ventricle failure and dilation

↑ Pulmonary blood pressure

Among the lung diseases capable of causing pulmonary hypertension are chronic pulmonary disorders characterized by bronchoalveolar changes with fibrosis and emphysema, in which the pulmonary capillary bed can be reduced by up to 50%. The marked reduction of the capillary bed leads to pulmonary hypertension. The latter can be induced by several mechanisms: diffuse interstitial fibrosis, inflammation around pulmonary capillaries with vascular lumen narrowing, and obstructive conditions leading to hypoxemia with reflex pulmonary vasoconstriction. In most cases, these mechanisms are combined and produce distortion, compression and occlusion of broad regions of the pulmonary vascular tree. This causes vasoconstriction of pulmonary resistance vessels as a result of alveolar hypoxia and arterial hypoxemia. Chronic obstructive pulmonary disease (COPD) –which includes chronic bronchitis and emphysema– as well as bronchial asthma and cystic fibrosis among other conditions, are chronic lung diseases that can cause cor pulmonale (2)(3).

COPD and pulmonary circulation

↑ Collagen and proteoglycans

Muscular artery

Smooth muscle proliferation

Intimal thickening

Chronic pulmonary disease

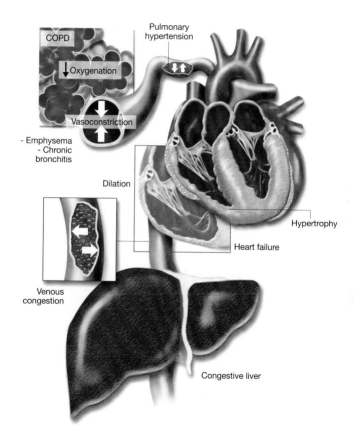

COPD

↓ Oxygenation

Vasoconstriction

- Emphysema
- Chronic bronchitis

Pulmonary hypertension

Dilation

Venous congestion

Hypertrophy

Heart failure

Congestive liver

Organic pulmonary insufficiency, whether congenital or acquired, is not a common disorder.

Instead, functional pulmonary insufficiency is more frequent since it is often secondary to pulmonary hypertension; also, it may result from mitral stenosis, chronic lung disease or pulmonary embolism. Incompetence is rarely related to structural valvular abnormalities. Valvular incompetence causes volume overload of the right ventricle and its progression depends on how the initial pulmonary hypertension is developed.

If it persists, the chronically overloaded ventricle becomes gradually dilated until insufficiency is eventually developed; this is referred to as cor pulmonale.

Diagnosis of these patients is made by auscultation of a mid-diastolic murmur in the pulmonary area, associated with signs of right ventricular hypertrophy.

Progression of patients with functional pulmonary regurgitation depends on the course of pulmonary hypertension (2)(3).

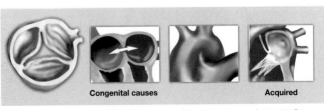

Congenital causes   **Acquired**

Interatrial   Patent ductus   Long-standing
communication   arteriosus   mitral stenosis

Valvular heart diseases: pulmonic regurgitation

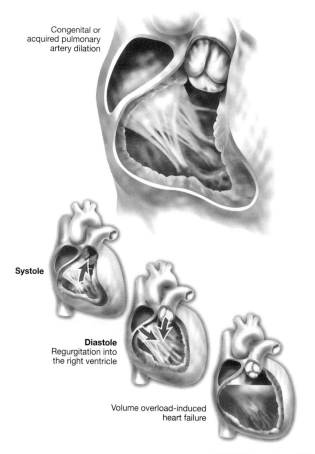

Congenital or acquired pulmonary artery dilation

Systole

Diastole
Regurgitation into the right ventricle

Volume overload-induced heart failure

Like in pulmonic regurgitation, organic tricuspid regurgitation is rare.
In most cases, there is functional regurgitation due to dilatation of
the valve ring in patients with right ventricular enlargement from any
cause. Symptoms of tricuspid regurgitation are the same as those
of pulmonary congestion and peripheral edema.

Hemodynamic compromise associated with tricuspid regurgitation
is largely dependent on the reflux produced to the superior and
inferior vena cavae as a result of valve incompetence.

It is at the hepatic level where clinical symptoms are more clearly
evidenced, on the one hand by a lift on palpation of the chest
produced by the beating of the enlarged right ventricle, and
a palpable thrill on the right hypochondrium during
ventricular systole.

The murmur is holosystolic along the left sternal border
and increases significantly during inspiration (2)(3).

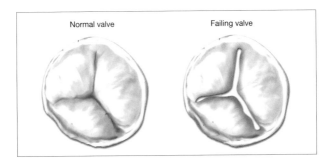

Normal valve   Failing valve

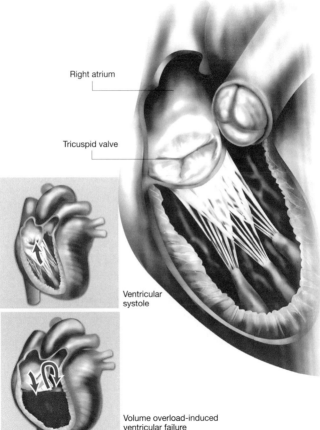

Right atrium

Tricuspid valve

Ventricular systole

Volume overload-induced ventricular failure

Right heart failure.
Clinical manifestations

When the right ventricle fails to pump enough blood to pulmonary circulation, the condition is referred to as right ventricular failure. Signs and symptoms related with this disorder occur in the areas of the body hemodynamically located behind the right ventricle, especially due to the stasis and venous hypertension produced in the territories of the superior and inferior vena cavae.

The most relevant manifestations are those associated with right ventricular backward failure:

• Venous engorgement: jugular engorgement is due to venous hypertension throughout the region above the atria.

• Edema: due to accumulation of fluids in body regions that slope downward, such as the ankles in standing people or the sacral region in bedridden patients.

• Painful hepatomegaly: venous congestion of the liver due to venous stasis in the inferior vena cava is evidenced by pain in right hypochondrium and diffuse, tender, smooth hepatomegaly.

• Effusions into cavities.

• Oliguria and nocturia: patients with right heart failure have reduced excretion of urine (oliguria); paradoxically, they also present with nocturia, due to edema reabsorption during the night (2)(3).

Right heart failure

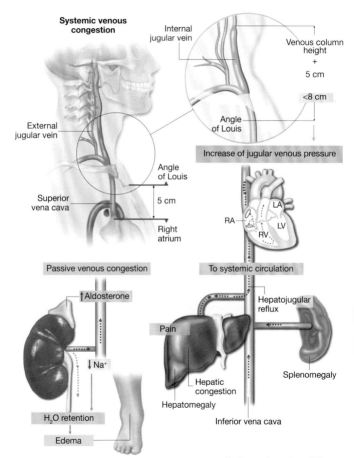

Systemic venous congestion

Internal jugular vein

Venous column height + 5 cm

<8 cm

Angle of Louis

External jugular vein

Angle of Louis

Superior vena cava

5 cm

Right atrium

Increase of jugular venous pressure

RA

LA

LV

RV

Passive venous congestion

↑Aldosterone

↓Na⁺

To systemic circulation

Hepatojugular reflux

Pain

Splenomegaly

H₂O retention

Hepatic congestion

Edema

Hepatomegaly

Inferior vena cava

Other causes of heart failure

Ischemic heart disease (IHD) results from an imbalance between myocardial oxygen supply and demand. In most cases, this imbalance is due to atherosclerosis of subepicardial coronary arteries. Coronary vasospasm, whether in isolation or associated with atherosclerosis, may contribute to reduced blood flow. Transmural myocardial infarction or multifocal areas of left ventricular necrosis can lead to an often fatal acute ischemic heart disease. On the contrary, long-standing ischemia results in diffuse myocardial atrophy and foci of scarring. In the long term, this progressively leads to CAD and congestive heart failure. These patients frequently develop angina pectoris with and without heart failure. On occasions, this already impaired cardiac reserve is abruptly exhausted upon an acute myocardial infarction. A recent infarction, even if small, can induce heart failure. In these circumstances, a healthy myocardial tissue is not sufficient –in spite of self-regulatory mechanisms– to achieve a minute volume adequate to meet the requirements of the body. Thus, it is not rare that an acute myocardial infarction is followed by acute left heart failure (2)(3).

**Right coronary artery
Frequent sites of obstruction**

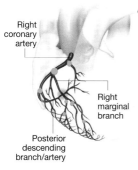

Right coronary artery

Right marginal branch

Posterior descending branch/artery

Impairment of the contractile function

Ventricular systole

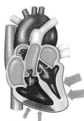

Akinetic area <56-78% of the volume

Left ventricle empties completely

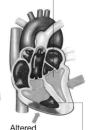

Altered inotropism

Damaged ventricle does not empty completely

**Left coronary artery
Frequent sites of obstruction**

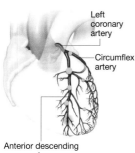

Left coronary artery

Circumflex artery

Anterior descending artery

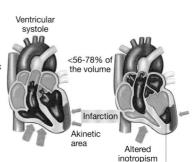

Ventricular systole

<56-78% of the volume

Infarction

Akinetic area

Altered inotropism

Ventricle does not empty completely

Any disorder or condition primarily affecting the myocardium and resulting in heart failure is called cardiomyopathy.

These conditions include infectious, metabolic and toxic cardiomyopathies, amyloidosis and endomyocardial fibrosis, among others.

Cardiomyopathies of unknown etiology are usually classified into hypertrophic (idiopathic hypertrophic subaortic stenosis or asymmetrical septal hypertrophy), dilated or congestive, and restrictive cardiomyopathies.

In the first type, the hypertrophied and excessively rigid muscle that cannot distend normally puts up resistance to ventricular filling, though systolic function is preserved until advanced stages. In dilated cardiomyopathies, there is myocardial dysfunction with reduced ejection fraction and increased end-systolic and end-diastolic volumes. Usually, there is global failure. In restrictive cardiomyopathies, there is inadequate ventricular filling during diastole due to decreased adaptability –similar to constrictive pericarditis– with early signs of congestive heart failure (2)(3).

Cardiomyopathies as a cause of heart failure

Types of cardiomyopathies		Chamber size	Ejection fraction	Ventricular pressure
Dilated	Biventricular dilation	⬆⬆	⬇⬇ Prone to failure	⬆⬆
Hypertrophied	Left ventricle and septal hypertrophy	Normal or ⬇	⬆⬆ Prone to dilated cardiomyopathy	Normal or ⬆
Restrictive	Impaired ventricular distensibility caused by infiltration	Normal or ⬆	Normal or ⬇ Prone to failure	⬆⬆
Obliterative	Endocardium thickened by mural thrombi	⬇	Normal or ⬇ Prone to failure	⬆

In this case, it is the myocardium itself that fails to pump blood after exhausting its adaptive mechanisms, including hypertrophy and ventricular dilation.

This intrinsic failure of the ventricular myocardium can be a primary failure in all those situations in which some process has caused muscle damage. For example, inflammation of the heart muscle or myocarditis. Although several microorganisms can cause myocardial inflammation, the most commonly involved ones are viral agents, such as Coxsackie virus, echovirus, and rubella, varicella and influenza viruses.

Viral myocarditis has a broad clinical spectrum. It may cause from sudden death, primarily among newborns and young infants, to a mild disease with apparently complete recovery. Between both ends, there is a great variety of clinical patterns, and it is not rare to find patients with a chronic evolution characterized by cardiomegaly with mitral regurgitation that progresses to congestive heart failure (2)(3).

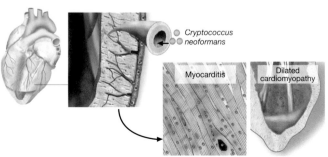

Cryptococcus neoformans

Myocarditis

Dilated cardiomyopathy

Myocarditis and heart failure

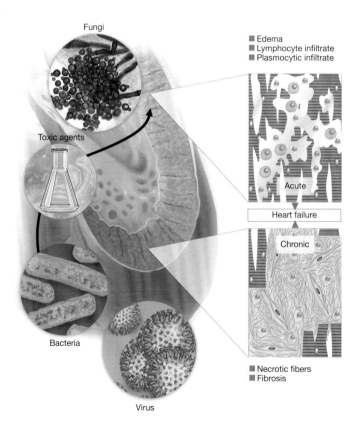

Fungi

Toxic agents

Bacteria

Virus

■ Edema
■ Lymphocyte infiltrate
■ Plasmocytic infiltrate

Acute

Heart failure

Chronic

■ Necrotic fibers
■ Fibrosis

In those patients in whom right ventricular involvement cannot be detected, the possibility of impaired ventricular filling is suspected, in most cases secondary to constrictive pericarditis. In constrictive pericarditis, a thickened fibrotic pericardium restricts expansion of the right chambers thus impairing normal diastolic filling.

A sudden accumulation of fluid in the pericardial cavity results in a marked increase of pericardial pressure due to poor pericardial distensibility. This affects right and left ventricular diastolic filling and alters systolic ejection to the aorta and pulmonary artery.

In acute cases, small volumes can cause cardiac tamponade, as it occurs in hemopericardium. Instead, if fluid accumulates gradually, the pericardium can tolerate larger amounts of fluid before developing disease. Clinically, there are signs of venous hypertension associated with others of hypotension.

The same as in cardiac tamponade, in constrictive pericarditis, a thickened fibrotic pericardium impedes cavity expansion thus impairing diastolic filling. In both cases, heart sounds are distant (2)(3).

Cardiac tamponade, constrictive pericarditis and heart failure

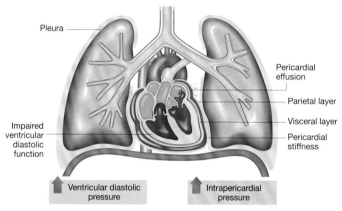

Pleura

Pericardial effusion

Parietal layer

Visceral layer

Pericardial stiffness

Impaired ventricular diastolic function

↑ Ventricular diastolic pressure

↑ Intrapericardial pressure

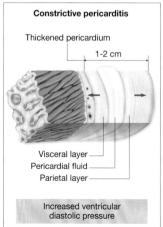

Constrictive pericarditis

Thickened pericardium

1-2 cm

Visceral layer
Pericardial fluid
Parietal layer

Increased ventricular diastolic pressure

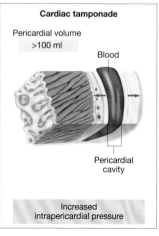

Cardiac tamponade

Pericardial volume >100 ml

Blood

Pericardial cavity

Increased intrapericardial pressure

Rheumatic heart disease results from cardiac involvement secondary to rheumatic fever. Clinical diagnosis of rheumatic fever is established by the presence of 2 major or 1 major and 2 minor manifestations included in the so-called "Jones criteria". If this diagnosis is supported by the evidence of a preceding streptococcal infection, the chances of having rheumatic fever are increased. The most severe manifestation of acute rheumatic fever is carditis since it can cause immediate death or chronic valvular damage. Clinically, patients have fever, organic murmur, tachycardia and signs of heart failure. Carditis can last some weeks up to several months and primarily affects the interstitial connective tissue in the proximity of blood vessels. After the initial attack, there are more chances of reactivation of the disease as a result of new streptococcal pharyngitis and probably every new reinfection will involve the same clinical findings. As a result of initial or subsequent attacks, patients can develop organic valvular heart disease usually involving the mitral and aortic valves. Valve stenosis, fibrosis, calcification, and deformity lead to permanent valve dysfunction and progressively cause severe heart failure, sometimes fatal after a few decades (2)(3).

Rheumatic fever and heart failure

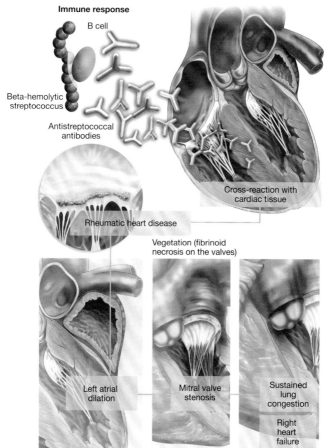

Immune response

B cell

Beta-hemolytic streptococcus

Antistreptococcal antibodies

Cross-reaction with cardiac tissue

Rheumatic heart disease

Vegetation (fibrinoid necrosis on the valves)

Left atrial dilation

Mitral valve stenosis

Sustained lung congestion

Right heart failure

Diseases of the venous system

Venous thrombi are intravascular deposits mainly consisting of fibrin and red blood cells, with a variable content of platelets and white blood cells.

Formation, growth and dissolution of venous thrombi reflect the balance between the effects of the thrombogenic stimulus and a number of protective mechanisms. Promoting factors include activation of blood clotting and venous stasis.

Vascular wall lesions are less important in the pathogenesis of venous thrombosis than in arterial thrombosis; however, in certain circumstances, they predispose to venous thrombosis.

Protective mechanisms include inactivation of clotting factors, dissolution and clearing of activated clotting factors, removal of the clotting factors activated by the liver, and fibrin dissolution by the fibrinolytic system.

Incidence of thromboembolism is higher among the elderly. Age itself is an independent risk factor; also, disorders with a proven thromboembolic risk are more frequent in this age group (37).

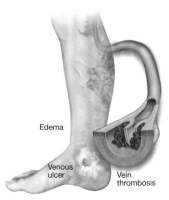

Edema

Venous
ulcer

Vein
thrombosis

Deep venous thrombosis

Promoting factors

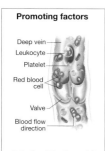

- Deep vein
- Leukocyte
- Platelet
- Red blood cell
- Valve
- Blood flow direction

- Activation of blood coagulation
- Venous stasis

Early phase

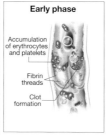

- Accumulation of erythrocytes and platelets
- Fibrin threads
- Clot formation

Final phase

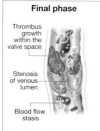

- Thrombus growth within the valve space
- Stenosis of venous lumen
- Blood flow stasis

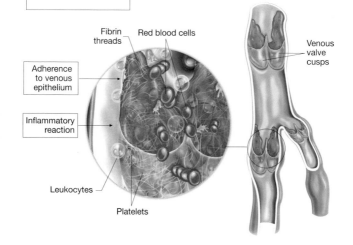

- Fibrin threads
- Red blood cells
- Adherence to venous epithelium
- Inflammatory reaction
- Leukocytes
- Platelets
- Venous valve cusps

Varicose veins appear as dilations of the superficial veins of the lower limbs.

In a standing position, the deep veins of the lower limbs receive a large blood volume that must flow back to the heart against gravity. The valvular system favors blood return to the heart.

When the valves of the deep system become incompetent, blood collects in collateral (communicating) veins and eventually passes to the superficial veins.

As these have a lower capacity, they cannot manage the excess blood volume normally, and dilate, giving rise to the so-called varicose veins.

A hypothesis has been proposed that varicose veins result from a congenital defect of the vein walls, more specifically, in the collagen.

Varicose veins are frequently associated with lower limb veins only, however, veins of any area of the body can be affected.

An example of this are the dilated veins of the hemorrhoidal plexus, which are referred to as hemorrhoids (37).

Varicose veins of the lower limbs

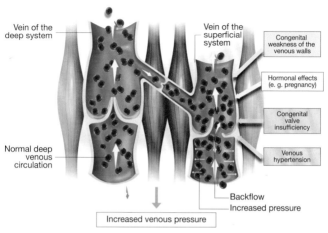

Vein of the deep system

Vein of the superficial system

Congenital weakness of the venous walls

Hormonal effects (e. g. pregnancy)

Congenital valve insufficiency

Venous hypertension

Normal deep venous circulation

Backflow

Increased pressure

Increased venous pressure

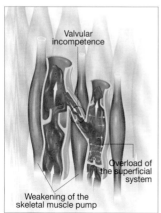

Valvular incompetence

Overload of the superficial system

Weakening of the skeletal muscle pump

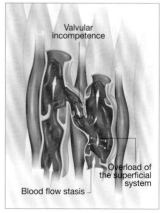

Valvular incompetence

Overload of the superficial system

Blood flow stasis

Once an acute episode of deep venous thrombosis (DVT) in the lower limbs has been overcome, the ideal circumstances may be met for the development of one of the most limiting processes that affect adults: symptomatic chronic venous insufficiency.

After a DVT episode including thrombus recanalization, the most affected is the valvular region, where irreversible lesions are sometimes described which impair future valve competence. Thus, backflow of blood is compromised resulting in collateral circulation via the perforator vessels to more superficial territories, giving rise to clinical expressions such as varicose veins and trophic lesions that range from hyperpigmentation to ulceration.

Location of the preceding deep venous thrombosis has been considered one of the most relevant factors to predict a post-thrombotic syndrome. Different authors have pointed out that involvement of popliteal and posterior tibial vessels is directly related with a greater predisposition. Likewise, the more proximal the lesion, the greater the likelihood that the syndrome develops (37).

Post-thrombotic syndrome

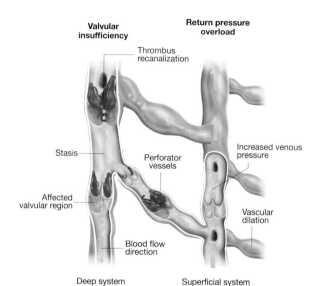

Valvular insufficiency

Return pressure overload

Thrombus recanalization

Stasis

Perforator vessels

Increased venous pressure

Affected valvular region

Vascular dilation

Blood flow direction

Deep system

Superficial system

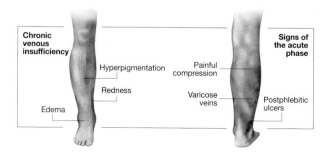

Chronic venous insufficiency

Signs of the acute phase

Hyperpigmentation

Painful compression

Redness

Varicose veins

Postphlebitic ulcers

Edema

The incidence of deep venous thrombosis (DVT) is very high in hospitalized patients. The most frequent location of venous thrombosis are the lower legs, where it is referred to as distal DVT. Next in frequency are the veins above the knee –femoropopliteal veins and then, the inferior vena cava and iliac veins–, where it is termed proximal DVT. The main cause of death in DVT is pulmonary embolism.

Although the clinical characteristics of pulmonary embolism are not specific, it may be suspected in patients with dyspnea, pleuritic pain, hemoptysis, tachypnea, etcetera.

Presumption of this disorder is increased in the presence of risk factors, when there is no other explanation for symptoms, and if there are signs of right heart failure.

Upon suspicion of pulmonary embolism, a ventilation-perfusion lung scan with a gamma camera should be performed; based on the results, which define the size and (mis)-matching of ventilation-perfusion defects, the probability of pulmonary embolism is obtained (37).

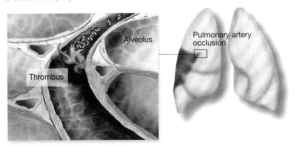

Alveolus

Pulmonary artery occlusion

Thrombus

Pulmonary thromboembolism

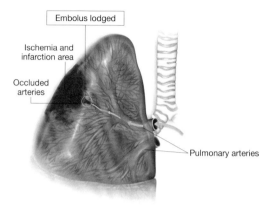

Embolus lodged

Ischemia and infarction area

Occluded arteries

Pulmonary arteries

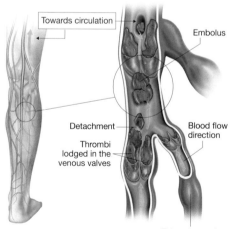

Towards circulation

Embolus

Detachment

Blood flow direction

Thrombi lodged in the venous valves

External granular appearance

Other cardiovascular diseases

One of the most noteworthy consequences of all the forms of vascular disease is aneurysm formation. An aneurysm is an abnormal local dilation of a blood vessel.

They are not rare and incidence usually increases with age. At least 10% of autopsies show aneurysms of the aorta and other arteries. Classification of aneurysms according to their macroscopic aspect is meant to describe their shape and size. Atherosclerotic aneurysms are usually located below the renal arteries and above the aortic bifurcation. Syphilitic aneurysms, instead, are typical of the thoracic aorta. The most common location for aneurysms is the abdominal aorta. Most abdominal aortic aneurysms are located below the renal arteries, sometimes extending into the common iliac arteries. This condition is most frequently observed in men over the age of 65, one of the most common contributing factors being atherosclerosis. If untreated, aneurysms naturally undergo progressive enlargement followed by rupture (3)(5)(9).

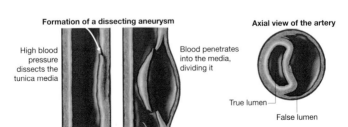

Formation of a dissecting aneurysm

High blood pressure dissects the tunica media

Blood penetrates into the media, dividing it

Axial view of the artery

True lumen

False lumen

Aneurysms. Macroscopic aspect and localization

Main location according to the cause

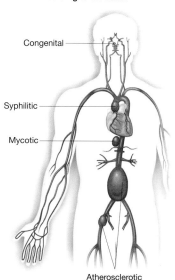

Congenital

Syphilitic

Mycotic

Atherosclerotic

Abdominal aortic aneurysm

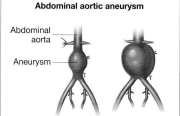

Abdominal aorta

Aneurysm

Different morphological aspects

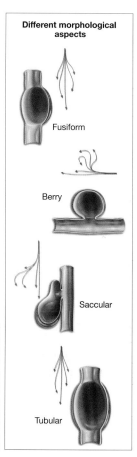

Fusiform

Berry

Saccular

Tubular

In the long term, diabetics can develop two types of vascular complications: microangiopathy and macroangiopathy (atherosclerosis). Initially, microangiopathy involves reversible functional impairment. Later in the disease, there are morphologic changes which can only be stabilized or reversed in the early stages by optimizing metabolic control. Frequency and severity of microangiopathy have some correlation with duration and control of diabetes. Although the mechanism of action is not fully understood, hyperglycemia is thought to play a central role.

Morphologically, diabetic microangiopathy is characterized by diffuse thickening of the capillary basement membrane, primarily in the skin, skeletal muscle, retina, renal glomerulus and renal medulla. In middle and large-sized vessels, diabetes enhances the extent and severity of atherosclerosis. Although it is rare to find significant atherosclerosis in healthy premenopausal women, diabetes promotes earlier development of the disease. In diabetic individuals, thrombotic occlusion of large and medium-sized atherosclerotic arteries is much more common. Thus, myocardial and cerebral infarction are very usual complications of this disease (38)(39).

Diabetic angiopathy

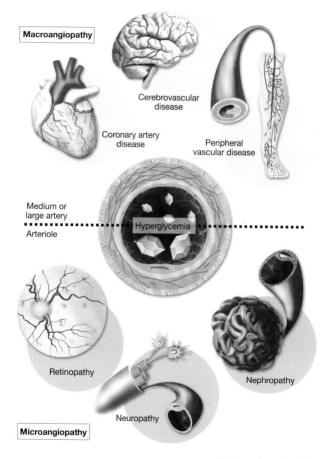

Macroangiopathy

Cerebrovascular disease

Coronary artery disease

Peripheral vascular disease

Medium or large artery

Arteriole

Hyperglycemia

Retinopathy

Neuropathy

Nephropathy

Microangiopathy

References

(1) Williams PL et al. Gray's Interactive Anatomy CD-ROM. 38va. edición. Elsevier Science, 1998.

(2) Guyton AC y Hall JE. Textbook of medical physiology. Philadelphia: WB Saunders, 2000.

(3) Bertolasi C, Barrero C y col. Cardiología 2000. Bs. As.: Ed. Médica Panamericana, 2001.

(4) Cingolani H, Houssay A y cols. Fisiología Humana. Bs. As.: El Ateneo, 2000.

(5) Braunwald E, Libby P, Zipes DP. Heart Disease: A Textbook of Cardiovascular Medicine, 6ta. edición. WB Saunders, 2001.

(6) Ganong W. Fisiología Médica, 14ta. edición. México D.F.: Manual Moderno, 1994.

(7) Farreras Valentín P, Roman C. Medicina Interna. 13° edición. Madrid: Harcourt Brace, 1997.

(8) Rubenstein E & Federman D. Medicine, 1ra. edición. New York: Scientific American, 1995.

(9) Contran Robbins. Patología estructural y funcional, 4ta. edición. Madrid: McGraw-Hill Interamericana, 1990.

(10) Esper R, Mazzei J. Biblioteca de Medicina: Cardiología. Bs. As.: El Ateneo, 1992.

(11) Third Report of the National Cholesterol Education Program (NCEP) Expert Panel on Detection, Evaluation, and Treatment of High Blood Cholesterol in Adults (Adult Treatment Panel III). Final Report. Circulation 2002;106:3143.

(12) Grundy SM, Cleeman JI, Bairey Merz CN y col. NCEP REPORT. Implications of Recent Clinical Trials for the National Cholesterol Education Program Adult Treatment Panel III Guidelines. Circulation 2004;110:227-39.

(13) Zaret BL, Moser M, Cohen LS. Yale University School of Medicine-Heart Book, Yale University, 1992.
www.info.med.yale.edu/library/heartbk/

(14) Coughlan BJ, Sorrentino MJ. Does hypertriglyceridemia increase risk for CAD?: growing evidence suggests it plays a role. Postgrad Med 2000;108(7): 77-84.

(15) Russell R. Atherosclerosis - An inflammatory disease. NEJM 1999;340(2):115-26.

(16) Sposito AC, Chapman MJ. Statin Therapy in Acute Coronary Syndromes. Arteriosclerosis, Thrombosis, and Vascular Biology 2002;22:1524.

(17) Hansson GK. Immune Mechanisms in Atherosclerosis. Arteriosclerosis, Thrombosis, and Vascular Biology 2001;21:1876.

(18) Kawashima S. Malfunction of Vascular Control in Lifestyle-Related Diseases: Endothelial Nitric Oxide (NO) Synthase / NO System in Atherosclerosis. J Pharmacol Sc 2004;96:411-19.

(19) Cai H, Harrison DG. Endothelial Dysfunction in Cardiovascular Diseases: The Role of Oxidant Stress. Circ.Res Nov 2000;87:840-44.

(20) Stary HC, Chandler B, Dinsmore RE. A Definition of Advanced Types of Atherosclerotic Lesions and a Histological Classification of Atherosclerosis. A Report From the Committee on Vascular Lesions of the Council on Arteriosclerosis, American Heart Association. Circulation 1995;92:1355-74.

(21) Grech ED. Pathophysiology and investigation of coronary artery disease. BMJ 2003;326: 1027-30.

(22) Jamshid Alaeddini, Behzad Alimohammadi. Angina pectoris. Last update, january 24, 2005.
http://www.emedicine.com/med/topic133.htm

(23) Parker JO. Angina Pectoris: A Review of Current and Emerging Therapies. Am J Manag Care 2004;10:S332-S338.

(24) Yeghiazarians Y, Braunstein JB, Askari A. Unstable Angina Pectoris. NEJM 2000;342(2): 101-114.

(25) Myocardial Infarction Redefined-A Consensus Document of The Joint European Society of Cardiology/American College of Cardiology. Committee for the Redefinition of Myocardial Infarction. The Joint European Society of Cardiology/American College

of Cardiology Committee European Heart Journal 2000;21:1502-13.

(26) Stahmer S. Myocardial Infarction. Last Updated: January 6, 2005.
http://www.emedicine.com/emerg/topic327.htm

(27) Zimetbaum PJ, Josephson ME. Use of the electrocardiogram in Acute Myocardial Infarction. NEJM 2003;348:933-40.

(28) Farb A, Tang AL, Burke AP y col. Sudden Coronary Death: Frequency of Active Coronary Lesions, Inactive Coronary Lesions, and Myocardial Infarction. Circulation Oct 1995;92:1701-09.

(29) Alpert y Thygesen et al. Myocardial infarction redefined. Journal of the American College of Cardiology 2000;36(3):959-969.

(30) Berger PB, Orford JL. Acute Myocardial Infarction. ACP Medicine 2004. American College of Physicians.
http://www.medscape.com/viewarticle/491020

(31) Golledge J, Greenhalgh RM, Davis A. The symptomatic carotid plaque. Stroke. 2000;31: 774.

(32) Victor M, Ropper AH, Adams RD. Adams & Victor Principles of Neurology, 7th. edition, McGraw-Hill Professional, 2000.

(33) Braunwald E, Fauci AS, Kasper DL and colls. Harrison's Principles of Internal Medicine, 15th. edition. McGraw-Hill Professional Publishing, 2001.

(34) Beard JD. Chronic lower limb ischaemia. British Medical Journal 2000;320: 854-57.

(35) Kelly WN. Medicina Interna, segunda edición. Bs. As.: Editorial Médica Panamericana, 1992.

(36) Mc Laughlin K, Jardine AG, Moss JC. Renal Artery Stenosis. British Medical Journal 2000; 320:1124-27.

(37) Ribera Casado JM, Cruz Jentoft AJ. Patología vascular periférica en geriatría. Masson S.A., Barcelona, 1998.

(38) Cecil. Textbook of Medicine, 21st. edition. Philadelphia: WB Saunders 2001.

(39) Noble. Textbook of Primary Care Medicine, 3ra. edición. Mosby, 2001.

Tables with laboratory reference range values and other data of interest

---

Specialized web sites

Chemical constituents of the blood *(International Units)*

Acetoacetate P	<100 µmol/litre	(5)
Ascorbic acid S	23-85 µmol/litre	(4)
Red cell folate	7-39.7 nmol/litre	(1)(4)(5)
Uric acid	150-480 µmol/litre	(1)(5)(6)
Albumin	35-55 grams/litre	(1)(4)(5)(6)
Alpha-1-antitrypsin	0.8-2.1 grams/litre	(1)
Alpha-2-macroglobulin	0.15-0.4 grams/litre	(1)
Alpha-fetoprotein	<15 µgrams/litre	(1)(5)
Ammonia	6-47 µmol/litre	(1)(4)
Antistreptolysin	<250 Todd units	(4)
Conjugated (direct) bilirubin	1.7-7.0 µmol/litre	(1)(4)(5)(6)
Unconjugated (indirect) bilirubin	3.4-12 µmol/litre	(1)(4)(5)(6)
Total bilirubin	5.1-17 µmol/litre	(1)(4)(5)(6)
Total calcium	2.2-2.6 mmol/litre	(1)(4)(5)(6)
Ionized calcium	1.1-1.4 mmol/litre	(1)(4)
Carotenoids	1.5-74 µmol/litre	(4)
CEA		
smokers	<0.5 ng/ml	(8)
non-smokers	<2.5 ng/ml	(8)
Ceruloplasmin	270-3 mg/litre	(1)
Zinc	12-30 µmol/litre	(4)
Copper	11-24 µmol/litre	(4)
Creatinine	35-105 µmol/litre	(4)(6)
Carbon dioxide (CO_2)	24-30 mmol/litre	(4)
Enzymes		
aldolase	0-6 U/litre	(1)
amylase	60-180 U/litre	(1)
creatine phosphokinase (CPK)	40-400 U/litre	(1)(5)
prostatic acid phosphatase (PAO)	<4 mU/ml	(1)(4)
alkaline phosphatase (Alk. Phos.)	40-129 U/litre	(1)(7)
gamma glutamyl transpeptidase	0.07-1 µmol/L (S)	(4)
lactate dehydrogenase (LDH)	750-1500 U/litre (S)	(5)
transaminases GOT or AST	5-32 mU/ml	(1)
transaminases GPT or ALT	7-33 mU/ml	(1)
5'-nucleotidase	0-11 U/litre	(1)(4)
Serum iron	9-27 µmol/litre	(4)
Ferritin	15-300 µg/litre	(4)(6)
Fibrinogen	1.5-4 grams/litre	(1)
Phospholipids	150-250 mg/dl	(1)
Inorganic phosphorus	0.7-1.4 mmol/litre	(4)(6)
GGT	0.07-1 mmol/L (S)	(4)
Globulins	23-35 grams/litre	(4)(6)
Blood glucose	3.9-6.4 mmol/litre	(1)(4)
Haptoglobin	27-139 mg/dl	(1)(4)

Chemical constituents of the blood (Cont.)

Fetal hemoglobin	<2%	(4)
Glycosylated hemoglobin	<5%	(4)
Serum hemoglobin	0.01–0.05 grams/litre	(5)
Iron	9-27 µmol/litre	(1)(4)(6)
Immunoglobulins		
IgA	1.4-2.9 grams/litre	(4)
IgD	0.003-0.040 grams/litre	(4)
IgE	0.001-0.003 grams/litre	(4)
IgG	9-15 grams/litre	(4)(6)
IgM	0.7-2.5 grams/litre	(4)
Lactate (lactic acid)	0.5-1.5 mmol/litre	(4)
Magnesium	0.8-1.3 mmol/litre	(4)
Methemoglobin	<1%	(4)
NaCl	96-106 mEq/L	(4)
Non-protein nitrogen (NPN)	15-35 mg/dl	(4)
Blood urea nitrogen (BUN)	0.8-3.3 mmol/litre	(4)(6)
Plasma osmolarity	280-300 mOsmol/L	(4)
C peptide	2.10 ± 0.54 ng/ml	(4)
Pyruvate	0-0.11 mmol/L	(4)
Potassium	3.5-5.0 mmol/litre	(4)(6)
Sodium	135-147 mmol/litre	(4)(6)
Transferrin	23-45 mmol/litre	(4)
Urea	1.7-6.7 mmol/litre	(4)

Complete blood count

Red blood cells

-men	$4.5x5.9x10^6$ cell/mm^3	(1)(2)(4)(6)
-women	4-5.2 cell/mm^3	(1)(2)(4)(6)
Hemoglobin		
-men	8.4-10.9 mmol/litre	(1)(2)(4)
-women	7.4-9.9 mmol/litre	(1)(2)(4)
Hematocrit		
-men	0.41-0.53	(1)(2)(4)(6)
-women	0.36-0.46	(1)(2)(4)(6)
Erythrocyte sedimentation rate		
-men	0-17 mm/hr	(5)
-women	1-25 mm/hr	(5)
Reticulocytes	0.5-20%	(2)(4)
Siderocytes	0.01-0.1%	(4)
MCH	29 ± 2 pg	(4)
MCHC	340 ± 2 grams/litre	(4)
MCV	90 ± 7 fl	(4)
Leucocytes	5000-10 000 cell/mm^3	(4)
Lymphocytes	17-45%	(4)

Complete blood count (Cont.)

Monocytes .... 2-8% .... (4)
Neutrophil band forms .... 0-6% .... (4)
Segmented neutrophils .... 55-70% .... (4)
Eosinophils .... 1-4% .... (4)
Platelets .... 150-350x10^9 plt/litre .... (5)

Coagulation

Antithrombin III .... 220-390 mg/litre .... (1)
Prothrombin consumption
   Prothrombin time (Quick) .... 12-14 sec .... (4)
   Thrombin time .... 15-20 sec .... (1)(4)
Capillary resistance (Rumpel-Leede method) .... <6 petechiae .... (4)
Clot retraction .... 50-100%/2hrs .... (4)
Coagulation time (Lee-White) .... 5-11 min .... (4)
Bleeding time
   Ivy .... 2.5-9.5 min .... (1)(4)(6)
   Duke .... 1-4 min .... (4)
Partial thromboplastin time (kPTT) .... <10 sec .... (4)

Hormone measurements in blood

11-deoxycortisol .... 0.34-4.56 nmol/litre ..... (1)(5)
17-β-estradiol
women:
-follicular phase .... 184-532 pmol/litre .... (1)(5)
-midcycle .... 411-1626 pmol/litre ..... (1)(5)
-luteal phase .... 184-885 pmol/litre .... (1)(5)
-postmenopausal .... 217 pmol/litre .... (1)(5)
men: .... 184 pmol/litre .... (1)(5)
ACTH (adrenocorticotropic hormone) .... 1.3-16.7 pmol/litre ...... (1)(5)
ADH (antidiuretic hormone) .... 2.4 ± 0.9 ng/litre .... (4)
Epinephrine (supine position) .... <273 pmol/litre .... (1)(5)
Aldosterone (supine position, normal diet) .... 55-250 pmol/litre .... (1)(5)
Androstenedione .... 1.75-8.73 nmol/litre ..... (1)(5)
Angiotensin II .... <25 pg/ml .... (4)
Calcitonin .... 0-28 pg/ml .... (4)
Cortisol .... 138-690 nmol/litre .... (1)(5)
DHEA
-men: .... 6.24-41.6 nmol/litre ..... (1)(5)
-women: .... 4.5-34.0 nmol/litre ...... (1)(5)
Dihydrotestosterone
-men: .... 1.03-2.92 nmol/litre ..... (1)
-women: .... 0.14-0.76 nmol/litre ..... (1)
DOCA (deoxycorticosterone) .... 61-576 nmol/litre .... (1)(5)
Dopamine .... <475 pmol/litre .... (1)(5)

Hormone measurements in blood (Cont.)

Estrone
women:
- follicular phase .... 55-555 pmol/litre .... (1)(5)
- luteinic phase .... 55-740 pmol/litre .... (1)(5)
- postmenopausal .... 55-204 pmol/litre .... (1)(5)
men .... 55-240 pmol/litre .... (1)(5)
FSH
women:
-follicular phase .... 3.0-20.0 IU/litre .... (1)(5)
-ovulation .... 9.0-26.0 IU/litre .... (1)(5)
-luteinic phase .... 1.0-12.0 IU/litre .... (1)(5)
-postmenopausal .... 18.0-153.0 IU/litre ... (1)(5)
men .... 1.0-12.0 IU/litre .... (1)(5)
Gastrin .... <100 ng/litre .... (1)(5)
Glucagon .... 20-100 ng/litre .... (1)(5)
Glucose .... 3.8-6.1 mmol/litre ..... (1)(6)
Human chorionic gonadotropin .... <5 IU/litre .... (5)
17-hydroxyprogesterone
 women:
-follicular phase .... 0.6-3.0 nmol/litre ...... (1)(5)
- ovulation .... 3.0-7.5 nmol/litre ...... (1)(5)
-luteal phase .... 3.0-15 nmol/litre .... (1)(5)
-postmenopausal .... ≤2.1 nmol/litre .... (1)(5)
men: .... 0.15 nmol/litre .... (1)(5)
Insulin .... 14.35-143.50 pmol/litre(1)(5)
LH
women:
-follicular phase .... 2.0-15.0 IU/litre .... (1)(5)
-ovulation .... 22.0-105.0 IU/litre .... (1)(5)
-luteal phase .... 0.6-19.0 IU/litre .... (1)(5)
-postmenopausal .... 16.0-64.0 IU/litre ..... (1)(5)
men: .... 2.0-12.0 IU/litre .... (1)(5)
Norepinephrine (supine position) .... 650-2423 pmol/litre .... (1)(5)
Parathormone .... 10-60 ng/litre .... (1)(5)
C peptide .... 0.17-0.66 nmol/litre .... (1)(5)
PRL
-men .... 0-15 µg/litre .... (1)(5)
-women .... 0-20 µg/litre .... (1)(5)
Progesterone
women:
-follicular phase .... <0.6 nmol/litre .... (1)(5)
-luteinic phase .... 9.54-63.6 nmol/litre .... (1)(5)
men: .... <0.60-4.45 nmol/litre ... (1)(5)
Renin (activity) .... 1.4 ± 0.92 ng/ml/h .... (4)

Hormone measurements in blood (Cont.)

Somatomedin C
  16-24 years .... 182-780 µg/litre .... (1)(5)
  25-39 years .... 114-492 µg/litre .... (1)(5)
  40-54 years .... 90-360 mg/litre .... (1)(5)
  >54 years .... 71-290 µg/litre .... (1)(5)
Somatostatin .... <25 ng/litre .... (1)(5)
STH .... 0.5-17.0 µg/litre .... (1)(5)
Free T_3 .... 0.22-6.78 pmol/litre ... (1)(5)
Total T_3 .... 0.92-2.78 nmol/litre ... (1)(5)
T_4 .... 58-155 nmol/litre .... (5)(6)
Free T_4 .... 10.3-35.0 pmol/litre .... (1)(5)
I123 uptake .... 8-30% of dose of I/24hs(6)
TSH .... 0.5-4.7 µg/litre .... (1)(5)
Testosterone
-women .... 0.21-2.98 nmol/litre ... (1)(5)
-men .... 9.36-37.10 nmol/litre ... (1)(5)

Arterial blood gases
pCO_2 .... 36-45 mm Hg .... (4)(6)
pH .... 7.37-7.45 .... (4)(6)
pO_2 .... 90-110 mm Hg .... (4)
Total plasma CO_2 .... 55-60 vol. % .... (4)
Oxyhemoglobin saturation .... 95-99% .... (4)
Bicarbonate .... 24-34 mEq/L .... (4)
Base excess .... +2.3/-2.3 mEq/L .... (4)

Protein electrophoresis
Albumin .... 35-55 grams/litre .... (1)(4)(5)(6)
Alpha 1 .... 2-4 grams/litre .... (1)
Alpha 2 .... 5-9 grams/litre .... (1)
Beta .... 6-11 grams/litre .... (1)
Gamma .... 7-17 grams/litre .... (1)
Globulins .... 20-35 grams/litre .... (1)
Total proteins .... 55-80 grams/litre .... (1)

Lipid profile
Desirable HDL cholesterol .... >1,55 mmol/litre .... (9)
Desirable LDL cholesterol .... <2,59 mmol/litre ....(9)
Desirable total cholesterol .... <5.17 mmol/litre ....(9)
Desirable triglycerides .... 0.45-1.69 mmol/litre ......(9)

Urine chemistry

17-ketosteroids .... 14-90 µmol/24 hr .... (4)
17-OH-corticosteroids .... 8-22 µmol/24 hr .... (4)(6)
Acetone .... negative .... (1)(4)(5)
Titratable acidity .... 20–40 mmol/24 hr .... (5)
Uric acid .... 1.49–4.76 mmol/24 hr ...... (5)
Vanillylmandelic acid .... 7.6–37.9 µmol/24 hr .... (5)
Epinephrine .... 4.3-30.9 mmol/day .... (4)
Albumin .... negative .... (1)(4)(5)
Amylase .... 4–400 U/litre .... (5)
Ammonia .... 30–50 mmol/24 hr .... (4)(5)
Calcium .... 2.5-7.5 mmol/24 hr .... (5)(6)
Chlorides
-Cl .... varies according to diet .... (6)
-NaCl .... varies according to diet .... (6)
Cortisol .... 55–193 nmol/24 hr .... (5)
Creatine (men) .... <380 µmol/24 hr .... (4)(5)
Creatine (women) .... <760 µmol/24 hr .... (4)(5)
Creatinine .... 0.13-0.22 mmol/kg/day ..... (1)(4)
Ketone bodies .... negative .... (1)(4)
Total estrogens .... 45-146 nmol/24 hr .... (6)
Phosphates .... 12.9–42.0 mmol/24 hr ...... (4)(5)
Glucose .... 0.3–1.7 mmol/24 hr .... (5)
Urea nitrogen .... 214–607 mmol/24 hr .... (5)
Osmolarity .... 300–900 mOsmol/kg .... (1)
Oxalates .... 228–684 µmol/24 hr .... (5)
pH .... 5.0–9.0 .... (1)(4)(5)
Porphyrins
  coproporphyrin .... 80-380 nmol/24hr .... (5)
  porphobilinogen .... negative .... (1)(4)(5)
Potassium .... 25–100 mmol/24 hr .... (5)
Proteins .... <0.15 g/24 hr .... (5)(6)
Sodium .... 100–260 mmol/24 hr .... (5)
Urea .... >10 g/litre .... (5)
Urobilinogen .... 1.7–5.9 µmol/24 hr .... (1)(5)

Vitamins

Vitamin A .... 0.7-3.5 nmol/L .... (1)(5)
Vitamin B_1 (thiamine) .... 0-75 nmol/L .... (1)(5)
Vitamin B_2 (riboflavin) .... 106-638 nmol/L .... (1)(5)
Vitamin B_6 .... 20-121 nmol/L .... (1)(5)
Vitamin B_{12} .... 148-590 pmol/L .... (1)(5)

Vitamins (Cont.)

Vitamin C (ascorbic acid)..................................... 23-57 µmol/L.................(1)(5)
Vitamin D$_3$ (1,25 dihydroxyvitamin D) .... 60-108 pmol/L ....(1)(5)
Vitamin D$_3$ (25 hydroxyvitamin D)........................ 37.4-200 nmol/L ....(1)(5)
Vitamin E... 12-42 µmol/litre ....(1)(5)
Vitamin K.. 0.29-2.64 nmol/L ....(1)(5)

Cerebrospinal fluid

Chlorides .... 120-130 mEq/L ....(3)(4)(6)
Proteins .... 15-30 mg/100 mL ......(3)(4)(6)
Albumin .... 10-30 mg/100 mL ......(3)(4)
Gammaglobulins .... 3-12% ....(3)(4)(6)
Glucose .... 50-80 mg/100 mL ......(3)(4)(6)
Pressure .... 10-20 cm/H$_2$0 (lying) ..(3)(4)
Cells (lymphocytes).. 0-5 number/mL ....(3)(4)(6)

Normal values of cardiovascular function

Heart rate .... 60-100 beats/minute... (4)
Blood pressure (humeral)...................................... 100-160 /60-90 mm Hg (4)
Venous pressure (cubital vein)............................. 7-12 cmH$_2$0 .... (4)
Intracardiac pressures
Pulmonary artery:
  systolic .... <30 mm Hg .... (4)
  diastolic.. <15 mm Hg .... (4)
  mean .... <20 mm Hg .... (4)
Pulmonary arteriolar-capillary (mean) .... <12 mm Hg .... (4)
Aorta.. 100-160/60-90 mm Hg (4)
Left auricle (mean)... <12 mm Hg .... (4)
Right auricle (mean) .... <5 mm Hg .... (4)
Left ventricle:
  systolic .... 100-160 mm Hg............ (4)
  diastolic 1... 0 mm Hg .... (4)
  diastolic 2 (telediastolic) .... <12 mm Hg .... (4)
Right ventricle:
  systolic .... <30 mm Hg .... (4)
  diastolic 1... 0 mm Hg .... (4)
  diastolic 2 (telediastolic) .... <5 mm Hg .... (4)

Renal function tests

Glomerular filtration rate
  Measured by inulin clearance .... 125-140 ml/min .... (4)
  Measured by endogenous creatinine .... 90-130 ml/min .... (4)
  clearance

Renal function tests (Cont.)

Renal plasma flow
    Measured by the clearance of .... 50-650 ml/min .... (4)
    para-aminohippuric acid
    Urea clearance.. 60-100 ml/min .... (4)
Concentration and dilution tests (urine specific gravity)........................
    maximum concentration after 12 hours .... 1.025 or higher............ (4)
    of water restriction and a dry diet
    maximum dilution after water .... 1.003 or lower.............. (4)
    overload of 1,000 mL

References
(1) Kasper DL, Braunwald E, Fauci A, Hauser S, Longo D, Jameson JL. Harrison's Principles of Internal Medicine. 16th. edition. McGraw-Hill Professional; July 23, 2004.
(2) Beers M, Berkow R. El manual Merk de diagnóstico y tratamiento. 10º edición española. Madrid: Ediciones Harcourt S. A. 1999.
(3) Kennet Walker H, Dallas Hall W, Willis Hurt J. Clinical Methods, The history, physical and laboratory examinations. 1990. Butterworth Publishers. http://www.ncbi.nlm.nih.gov/books/bv.fcgi?rid=cm
(4) Farreras Valenti P, Rozman C. Medicina Interna. 14º edición. Harcourt Brance, 2000.
(5) Kratz A, Ferraro M, Sluss, Lewandrowski KB, Laboratory Reference Values. N Engl J Med 2004; 351: 1548-63.
(6) Telser A. Laboratory values Northwestern University Medical. http://www.galter.northwestern.edu/reftools/normals.html
(7) García Unzueta MT. Determinaciones analíticas: calcio, fósforo, fosfatasa alcalina, parathormona, vitamina D. http://departamentos.unican.es/med&psiq/MI/Capitulo%2012.pdf
(8) Dtsch MB. Colon carcinoma. Preoperative CEA, tumor differentiation and prognosis. Wochenschr, 1987 Aug 14;112(33):1245-9.
(9) Third Report of the National Cholesterol Education Program (NCEP) Expert Panel on Detection, Evaluation, and Treatment of High Blood Cholesterol in Adults (Adult Treatment Panel III). Final Report. National Institutes of Health. National Heart, Lung and Blood Institute. NIH Publication No. 02-5215. September 2002.

Essential nutrients and source food

Essential nutrient	Source food
Vitamin A (retinol)	As provitamin A (ß-carotene): in orange fruits and dark green vegetables. As retinol: fish liver oil, egg yolk, fortified dairy products
Vitamin D (cholecalciferol)	Fortified dairy, egg yolk, liver, fish liver oil; but the main source is exposure to ultraviolet rays
Vitamin E (α-tocopherol & other tocopherols)	Vegetable oils, vegetable margarine, wheat germ, leafy vegetables, beans
Vitamin K group (phylloquinone & menaquinone)	Cabbage, cauliflower, green leafy vegetables, egg yolk, liver. Vitamin K_2 synthesized by saprophyte intestinal flora
Vitamin B_1 Thiamin	Brewer´s yeast, meat, whole grains, dried fruit, beans, fortified cereal
Vitamin B_2 Riboflavin	Dairy productos, liver, meat, eggs, enriched cereal
Niacin	Brewer´s yeast, liver, fish, beans, whole grains, fortified cereal
Vitamin B_6 group (pyridoxine, pyridoxal, pyridoxamine)	Brewer´s yeast, entrails, cereal grains, beans, fish
Vitamin B_7 Biotin	Liver, kidney, egg yolk, cauliflower, yeast, dried fruit
Folic acid	Fresh green leafy vegetables, fruit, liver, yeast
Vitamin B_{12} (cobalamin)	Egg, meat, dairy (only animal products)
Vitamin C (ascorbic acid)	Citrus, kiwi, strawberries, tomatoes, cabbage, green pepper
Calcium	Milk and dairy productos, beans, cereal, meat
Zinc	Oysters, meat, liver, egg, cereal, peanuts
Chlorine	Widespread: basically, table salt
Copper	Dried fruit, oysters, pulses, entrails

Essential nutrients and source food (cont.)

Essential nutrient	Source food
Chromium	Yeast, liver, processed meat, cereal grains, spices
Phosphorous	Mild and dairy products, fish, poultry, meat, cereal, beans
Fluoride	Fish products, vegetables, cereals, coffee, tea, fluoride water
Iron	Meat, entrails, bivalve mollusks, soy beans, spinach.
	Only the iron contained in the meat "heme" group has good bioavailability (10-30% absorption)
Magnesium	Green leafy vegetables, cereal, dried fruit, fish products
Manganese	Cereal grains, leafy vegetables, dried fruit, tea
Molybdenum	Milk, beans, bread, cereal
Potassium	Milk, bananas, plums, raisins, meat
Selenium	Meat and animal products in general. Vegetables, according to the growing soil
Sodium	Table salt, packed and manufactured products in general
Iodine	Iodised salt, fish products, dairy products

Cytokines

Cytokine-Origin Interleukin (IL)	Main effects
IL-α IL-β: monocytes, macrophages	→ Pyrogen endogenous, sleep, anorexia, lymphocyte activation, IL-6 and CSF production
IL-2: T lymphocytes	→ Stimulates B and T cell growth, increases NK cell number
IL-3 : T lymphocytes, mast cells	→ Induces growth of hemopoietic progenitor cells
IL-4: T lymphocytes, mast cells	→ Stimulates T and B cell proliferation, IgE and IgE4 production, CD23 expression and release
IL-5: T lymphocytes, mast cells	→ Eosinophil differentiation. Stimulates IgA production

Cytokines (cont.)

IL-6: monocytes, fibroblasts, T lymphocytes
→ Pyrogen, production of acute phase protein, hematopoietic cell growth

IL-7: thymus, bone marrow
→ Induces proliferation of pro and pre B cells and immature thymocytes

IL-8: monocytes, endothelial cells, alveolar macrophages
→ Induces chemotaxis, T cell and neutrophil activation

IL-9: T lymphocytes
→ Proliferation of some T lymphocytes

IL-10: T lymphocytes, activated B lymphocytes and monocytes
→ Reduces MHC class II and antigenic presentation, stimulates B cell proliferation

IL-11: hematopoietic microenvironment
→ Proliferation of megacariocyte, macrophage progenitors proliferation

IL-12: monocytes, macrophages some mast cells and B cells
→ Inhibits IL-4, induces IgE and IFN-γ secretion

IL-13: B cells and macrophages
→ IgE secretion

IL-14: T cells
→ Stimulates B cell growth factor production

IL-15: muscle, non lymphoid cells
→ NK cell growth and cytotoxicity

IL-16: T cells
→ Increases MHC class II, suppresses HIV transcription

IL-17: CD4 cells
→ G-CSF secretion by endothelium, fibroblast production

Interferons (IFN)

IFN-α: leukocytes
→ Inhibits tumor growth and viral replication, increases NK cells

IFN-ß: fibroblasts
→ Same activity as above

IFN-γ: T cells T, NK cells
→ Macrophage activation, increases of MCH and II classes

Tumor Necrosis Factor (TNF)

TNF-α or cachectin: macrophages, monocytes
→ Increases IL, induces cytotoxic/cytostatic effects of GM-CSF, IFN-γ secretion

TNF-ß o lymphotoxin: T lymphocytes
→ Cytotoxic factor

Transforming Growth Factor (TGF)

TGF-α: carcinomas, sarcomas, monocytes
→ Stimulates angiogenesis, proliferation of keratinocytes, bone resorption, tumor growth

TGF-ß: platelets, B and T cells, placenta, kidney
→ Collagen and fibronectin synthesis, fibroblast proliferation, inhibits cell B and T proliferation

Chemokines

C: activated CD8, mast cells
→ Chemotaxis of T and NK cells

C-C
→ Idem above

C-X-C
→ Chemotaxis of T cells, mast cells, monocytes, eosinophils

C-X3-C
→ Not known exactly

Colony Stimulating Factor (CSF)

GM-CSF: T cells, monocytes, macrophages, endothelial cells
→ Induces growth of granulocyte and macrophage colonies, leukotriene production

G-CSF: monocytes, fibroblasts, endothelial cells
→ Induces granulocyte growth

M-CSF: idem above
→ Induces monocyte growth

Specialized web sites

American Board of Thoracic Surgery
http://www.abts.org/

American College of Cardiology
http://www.acc.org/

American Heart Association
http://www.americanheart.org/

American Heart Journal
http://www.harcourthealth.com/scripts/om.dll/
serve?action=searchDB&searchDBfor=home&id=hj

American Medical Association
http://www.ama-assn.org/

American Society for Microbiology
http://www.asm.org/

American Society of Echocardiography
http://asecho.org/

American Society of Hypertension
http://www.ash-us.org/

Angioplasty PTCA
http://www.ptca.org/

Asociación Venezolana de Aterosclerosis
http://www.geocities.com/HotSprings/Falls/2467/

Atlas of Myocardial Perfusion SPECT
http://brighamrad.harvard.edu/education/online/Cardiac/Cardiac.html

Australian Atherosclerosis Society
http://www.athero.org.au/default.htm

British Cardiac Society
http://www.bcs.com/

British Heart Foundation
http://www.bhf.org.uk/

British Medical Journal
http://www.bmj.com/

Canadian Cardiovascular Society
http://www.ccs.ca/

European Association for Cardio-thoracic Surgery
http://www.eacts.org/

European Atherosclerosis Society
http://www.elsevier.nl/homepage/sab/eas/

European Society for Vascular Surgery
http://www.esvs.org

European Society of Cardiology
http://www.escardio.org/

Food and Drug Administration (FDA)
http://www.fda.gov/

Fundación InterAmericana del Corazón
http://www.iahf.org/

Heart Failure Society of America
http://www.hfsa.org/

Heart Information Network
http://www.heartinfo.org/

International Society for Cardiovascular Surgery
http://www.vascularweb.org/

International Society for Heart Research
http://www.usouthal.edu/ishr/

Introduction to Cardiothoracic Imaging
http://info.med.yale.edu/intmed/cardio/imaging/

JAMA
http://jama.ama-assn.org/

North American Society for Cardiac Imaging
http://www.nasci.org/

PubMed
http://www.ncbi.nlm.nih.gov/PubMed/

Sociedad Española de Cardiología
http://www.secardiologia.es/

Sociedad InterAmericana de Hipertensión
http://www.musc.edu/iash/iashs.htm

Sociedad Latinoamericana de Cardiología Intervencionista
http://www.solaci.org/

Society of Cardiovascular & Interventional Radiology
http://www.scvir.org/

The Lancet
http://www.thelancet.com/

The New England Journal of Medicine
http://content.nejm.org/

The Society for Cardiac Angiography and Interventions
http://www.scai.org/

World Health Organization
http://www.who.int/home-page/

World Heart Federation
http://www.worldheart.org/

World Hypertension League
http://www.mco.edu/whl/index.html